Green Exercise

The concept of Green Exercise has now been widely adopted and implies a synergistic health benefit of being active in the presence of nature. This book provides a balanced overview and synthesis text on all aspects of Green Exercise and integrates evidence from many different disciplines including physiology, ecology, psychology, sociology and the environmental sciences, and across a wide range of countries.

It describes the impact of Green Exercise on human health and well-being through all stages of the life course and covers a wide spectrum from cellular processes such as immune function through to facilitating human behavioural change. It demonstrates the value of Green Exercise for activity and education purposes in both schools and the workplace, as well as its therapeutic properties. Green Exercise is an effective intervention for vulnerable groups and promoting healthy ageing, with activities including wilderness therapy, therapeutic horticulture and the use of forests and water. Chapters also integrate cross-cutting key themes which are relevant to all stages of the life course and have significantly contributed to the Green Exercise research base, such as forest bathing and blue exercise.

The book also explores the future of Green Exercise, the way in which research can be used to influence green design and planning and how health, social care and environmental agendas can be integrated to enable Green Exercise to be more widely used as a mechanism for improving health.

Jo Barton is Lecturer in Sports and Exercise Science at the University of Essex, UK.

Rachel Bragg is at Care Farming UK, and Visiting Fellow, University of Essex, UK.

Carly Wood is Lecturer in Nutrition and Exercise Science at the University of Westminster, London, UK.

Jules Pretty OBE is Professor of Environment and Society and Deputy Vice-Chancellor at the University of Essex, UK.

"Physical activity promotes health. Nature contact promotes health. This wonderful book explores the intersection of the two, providing both theory and evidence, across cultures, on the benefits of green exercise. It's timely, thorough, and readable – the definitive source on green exercise. Highly recommended."

– Howard Frumkin, School of Public Health,
University of Washington, USA

Green Exercise

Linking nature, health and well-being

Edited by Jo Barton, Rachel Bragg, Carly Wood and Jules Pretty

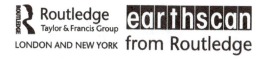

Routledge
Taylor & Francis Group

earthscan
from Routledge

LONDON AND NEW YORK

First published 2016
by Routledge
2 Park Square, Milton Park, Abingdon, Oxon OX14 4RN

and by Routledge
711 Third Avenue, New York, NY 10017

Routledge is an imprint of the Taylor & Francis Group, an informa business

British Library Cataloguing-in-Publication Data
A catalogue record for this book is available from the British Library

Library of Congress Cataloging in Publication Data
Names: Barton, Jo, editor.
Title: Green exercise : linking nature, health and well-being / edited by
Jo Barton, Rachel Bragg, Carly Wood and Jules Pretty.
Description: London ; New York : Routledge is an imprint of the
Taylor & Francis Group, an Informa Business, [2016] | Includes
bibliographical references and index.
Identifiers: LCCN 2015049599| ISBN 9781138807648 (hbk) | ISBN
9781138807655 (pbk) | ISBN 9781315750941 (ebk)
Subjects: LCSH: Exercise--Psychological aspects. | Nature--
Psychological aspects. | Outdoor recreation--Psychological aspects. |
Well-being. | Nature, Healing power of.
Classification: LCC GV706.4 .G736 2016 | DDC 613.7/1--dc23
LC record available at http://lccn.loc.gov/2015049599

ISBN: 978-1-138-80764-8 (hbk)
ISBN: 978-1-138-80765-5 (pbk)
ISBN: 978-1-315-75094-1 (ebk)

Typeset in Goudy
by HWA Text and Data Management, London

Contents

Figures and tables

Figures

Tables

Contributors

Bianca Ambrose-Oji, Social Scientist, Social and Economic Research Group, Forest Research, UK.

Jennie Aronsson, Lecturer in Adult Nursing, Plymouth University, UK.

Jo Barton, Lecturer in Sports and Exercise Science, and Member of Green Exercise Research Group, School of Biological Sciences, University of Essex, UK.

Sarah Bell, Associate Research Fellow, European Centre for Environment and Human Health, University of Exeter Medical School, UK.

Rachel Bragg, Development Coordinator at Care Farming UK and Visiting Fellow, University of Essex, UK.

Daniel Brown, Science Teacher, Stanway Federation Academy Trust, UK.

Maria Clark, Lecturer in Nursing, College of Medical and Dental Sciences, University of Birmingham.

Michael H. Depledge, Chair of Environment and Human Health, European Centre for Environment and Human Health, University of Exeter Medical School, UK and Visiting Professor at the Department of Zoology, Oxford University and at University College London.

Jason Duvall, Lecturer, Program in the Environment, University of Michigan, USA.

Lewis R. Elliott, PhD Student, European Centre for Environment and Human Health, University of Exeter Medical School, UK.

Helen Elsey, Lecturer in Public Health, Academic Unit of Public Health, Leeds Institute of Health Sciences, University of Leeds, UK.

Valerie Gladwell, Senior Lecturer in Sports and Exercise Science and Member of Green Exercise Research Group, School of Biological Sciences, University of Essex, UK.

Rochelle Gold, Research Manager, West Yorkshire Community Rehabilitation Company, Wakefield, UK.

Claire Henderson-Wilson, Senior Lecturer, Faculty of Health, Deakin University, Australia.

Rebecca Jenkin, PhD Student, European Centre for Environment and Human Health, University of Exeter Medical School, UK.

Stephen R. Kellert, Tweedy Ordway Professor Emeritus of Social Ecology and Senior Research Scholar, Yale School of Forestry and Environmental Studies, Yale University, USA.

Qing Li, President of the Japanese Society of Forest Medicine and Associate Professor, Department of Hygiene and Public Health, Nippon Medical School, Tokyo, Japan.

Neil Mapes, Managing Director, Dementia Adventure, UK.

Jenni Murray, Senior Research Fellow, Academic Unit of Public Health, Leeds Institute of Health Sciences, University of Leeds, UK.

Liz O'Brien, Head of Social and Economic Research Group, Forest Research, UK.

David Pencheon, Director, NHS/Public Health England Sustainable Development Unit, Cambridge, UK.

Jules Pretty, OBE, Professor of Environment and Society, School of Biological Sciences, Member of Green Exercise Research Group and Deputy Vice-Chancellor, University of Essex, UK.

Jo Roberts, CEO, Wilderness Foundation, UK.

Mike Rogerson, Research Officer and PhD Research Fellow (Sport and Exercise Sciences), Member of Green Exercise Research Group, School of Biological Sciences, University of Essex, UK.

Joe Sempik, Independent Research Consultant, UK.

William C. Sullivan, Professor and Head of Landscape Architecture, University of Illinois at Urbana-Champaign, USA.

Mardie Townsend, Honorary Associate Professor, Faculty of Health, Deakin University, Australia.

Sue Waite, Reader in Outdoor Learning, Plymouth Institute of Education, Plymouth University, UK.

Benedict W. Wheeler, Senior Research Fellow, European Centre for Environment and Human Health, University of Exeter Medical School, UK.

Mathew P. White, Senior Lecturer in Risk and Health, European Centre for Environment and Human Health, University of Exeter Medical School, UK.

Carly Wood, Lecturer in Nutrition and Exercise Science, Department of Life Sciences, University of Westminster, London, UK.

Preface

Jo Barton and Jules Pretty

Affluent countries and social groups across the world are facing a number of relatively new health and wellbeing challenges. Many of these are chronic non-communicable diseases and conditions that are lifestyle-driven, and include type 2 diabetes, obesity, cardiovascular disease, hypertension and some cancers. Many are a consequence of rising inactivity and rapid changes in food and calorie consumption, all of which also link to wider social changes and centre on shifting family and community structures, changing work and non-work opportunities, new transport options, and a demographic shift towards the elderly in populations. At the same time, natural environments worldwide continue to come under pressure – from urban and transport development, from climate change, and from the direct negative externalities of growth, such as air and water pollution.

Inactivity is now the fourth leading risk factor for mortality worldwide and is contributing to a rapidly growing financial burden on health services. Yet we also know that higher rates of physical activity and lower incidence of obesity have been associated with regular physical activity, time spent outdoors, and access to green space. It has become clear that the structure of environments, both social and natural, plays a role in encouraging active and healthy behaviours. Individuals with easy physical and cultural access to natural settings are three times as likely to engage in physical activity, experience less mental distress and have overall better wellbeing. In contrast, as residential distance from green space increases, the likelihood of being sufficiently physically active to prevent ill-health diminishes. The odds of becoming overweight or obese also significantly increase. Access to green space also improves perceived general health, reduces asthma prevalence, and risk of mental illness and stress levels, lowers morbidity and cardiovascular disease risk, increases life longevity, improves cognitive function and produces healthier cortisol profiles. We also know that people with green space close to their homes are less lonely, have more social support and experience an increased sense of community. Urban living has now become more common than rural worldwide, yet urban dwellers are more likely to develop mental illness, suffer from anxiety and develop mood disorders.

This book draws together internationally-recognised research on the synergistic health benefits of being physically active in green spaces: we call this *Green*

Exercise. We know both exercise and nature are independently facilitative of good health and wellbeing. The findings of recent research and practice suggest that the combination has an even more compelling effect. This book discusses the green exercise concept and brings together issues and research from a wide variety of disciplines from physiology through to environmental design. Novel perspectives cover the spectrum of health benefits from cellular to behavioural change, and the impacts of a variety of natural environments on health outcomes are assessed, including USA and UK urban nature, Australian parks, UK coastal settings and wildlands, and Japanese forests. We also consider the evidence for the benefits on a wide range of different social groups, and integrate cross-cutting key themes relevant to each stage of the life course from childhood to healthy ageing.

We also present the therapeutic properties of green exercise, known as *Green Care*, and present the outcomes of deliberate use of structured therapeutic programmes using walking, gardening and/or farming for vulnerable groups. Several chapters analyse the effectiveness of nature-based interventions for youth at risk, the role of probation services working from correctional facilities, individuals suffering from dementia, and the potential roles of green exercise in promoting healthier workforces. Some authors also explore how green exercise evidence could be used to influence urban design and planning, and how health and environmental agendas could be integrated to enable green exercise to be more widely used as a mechanism for both improving population health and maintaining natural environments.

We begin by discussing how environmental and social contexts shape health and wellbeing. Evidence is summarised to support seven interconnected themes that date back to the classical era of Asclepian healing. These feed directly into a number of chapters throughout the book. Nature contact is not only a multisensory experience, exposing individuals to sunlight to aid vitamin D production, but it also provides a space to be active, mindful, socially-interactive and to develop a sense of place and attachments to both people and places. Authors conclude it is important to incorporate nature into the design of buildings, hospitals, homes and community spaces to create shared spaces which facilitate interaction and attachment and increase opportunities for green exercise. This includes both direct experience of nature (for green exercise) and indirectly via paintings, pictures and views from the window. This evidence also calls for an integrated biophilic design of healthcare facilities to promote a nature experience that we know contributes to patient recovery and comfort and enhances performance and productivity of healthcare personnel. All too often, however, simple design principles are forgotten during urban development and building design. We conclude that investing in natural environments in all contexts equates to investing in human health and wellbeing.

Another key message of the book relates to the idea of an optimal dose of nature and green exercise for greatest health benefit. A dose of nature has been shown to have an immediate positive effect on mental health for a wide range of activities (e.g. walking, angling, cycling, gardening), for all age groups, for men and women, for every green environment and habitat (with additional benefits from the presence of water), and for the already healthy and the mentally-ill. However, identifying optimal doses needs to account for a wide range of mediators that include environmental factors such as quality (e.g. biodiversity, air quality, noise) and quantity (e.g. tree canopy cover) and weather; personal factors such as age, gender, beliefs about the value of nature, nature relatedness, prior experiences and childhood memories, as well as perceptions of risk; social and community factors including social interaction, trust, ethnic, cultural and social norms, and accessibility of green spaces.

For a variety of reasons, time spent outdoors appears to be diminishing, especially in affluent countries, so unplanned contact with nature occurs less often. Advances in technology and increased accessibility to computers and communication devices at a much earlier age may mean children are less likely to engage in outdoor play and recreation. Children today often learn more about the environment and nature from television and the internet than from real experience. This is despite mounting evidence that contact with nature has positive effects on physical and mental health, emotional and cognitive development, mental resilience, personal and social development, social skills and even academic achievements and life pathways. Unplanned outdoor activity helps encourage children to engage in spontaneous and unregulated play. Now disconnection is common. Using the outdoors as a learning space can help address this growing disconnection, making a strong argument for outdoor learning to be embedded in educational curricula: we know that active experiential learning in an alternative context enhances academic attainment, concentration and attention. Nature is thus also a learning resource that promotes resilience in young people and positively affects their future lifecourse opportunities.

It is not just green space that is of importance to health: blue environments by rivers, lakes and coasts seem to have intrinsic qualities that promote restoration and improved mental health and wellbeing. Authors also discuss evidence from coastal areas highlighting the importance of water for facilitating nature-based activities. Forests and woodlands also provide spaces for physical activity: research from Japan is leading the way in understanding and promoting forest bathing. Research shows walking in forests, forest bathing, reduces blood pressure and salivary cortisol, with greatest benefits shown for the elderly and those already with high blood pressure and more stress markers (again suggesting a therapeutic application). Further chapters discuss care farming as an intervention for probationers, the success of wilderness walking for youth at risk, and using nature to help those suffering from dementia to control and push back symptoms. Nature-based interventions offer a diverse applicability for many different cohorts of people and cumulatively this evidence should inform public health funding and government health and social care policies. Green exercise can be used as a vehicle to drive behavioural change and ensure a more inclusive approach to health.

The rise in inactivity levels and the associated problems with body-weight are a priority on many governments' agendas and although there is a general acknowledgement that green spaces encourage physical activity, the relationship between accessibility and health outcomes still needs further investigation. There are many areas of policy reform that could help increase the uptake of green exercise, though it is clear that there is a need for more detailed and comprehensive economic analyses to indicate exactly what benefits green exercise can bring to the whole economy. Participating in green exercise seems to be a more sustainable option in maintaining long-term activity levels. It is the interaction with the environment and the social contact that are the main incentives and the health benefits derived from the exercise are often secondary outcomes. Thus, competently managed, high-quality, accessible green spaces are essential for long-term sustainability and healthy communities. Green spaces offer collective benefits, but full economic costings need to be conducted. These would highlight the potential savings for national health systems and add further credence to the argument, attract national interest and set objectives for policy development.

In affluent countries, people have become more stressed, are more likely to experience mental ill-health, are at higher risk of developing non-communicable diseases, and are less active and more sedentary. Green exercise offers one way of addressing these emerging health problems successfully, quickly and cost-effectively. This book offers some potential solutions. It contains diverse international evidence from around the world on the health benefits of green exercise and nature-based interventions. The type of nature, activities, cultures and individuals may all vary but the message is universal and clear: green exercise benefits individual health and wellbeing, increases knowledge and care for natural environments, and provides a policy link between health and the environment.

Chapter 1

The seven heresies of Asclepius

How environmental and social context shapes health and well-being

Jules Pretty and David Pencheon

Well-being in modern societies

Asclepius was the Greek god of healing and medicine. From the 6th century BCE, some 800 Asclepian healing temples were built across the eastern and central Mediterranean. Typically, these were situated far from settlements on hilltops and promontories overlooking the sea, such as at Epidaurus, Pergamon and Kos, where light was multidirectional from sky and water, winds plentiful, and aromatics from pine forests and thyme-rich garrigue filled the air. At that time, it was assumed that well-being emerged from natural places (Hart, 1965; Gesler, 1993; Koenig, 2000). It is now increasingly being recognised that the natural and social context of individuals is a key determinant of well-being, providing protection against stressors and improving resilience and recovery (Sternberg, 2009; NEA, 2011).

The past century has seen great advances in health care and treatment. Mortality rates have fallen in most countries, and average lifespans are extending. Since the mid-1960s, mean life expectancy worldwide has risen from 56.0 to 70.4 years, and under-5 mortality has fallen sharply from 153 to 52 per 1000 live births; in the UK, under-5 mortality has fallen from 22 to 5 per 1000 (UNICEF, 2012). Over the same period, however, a new wave of health and well-being problems in modern societies has emerged largely as a result of changing lifestyles and the environments that shape these lifestyles (CMO, 2013).

Affluent societies are characterised by high levels of material consumption, abundant food and calories, a lower incidence of regular physical activity (increased sedentariness), a shifting demographic with a growing proportion of elderly people with care needs and often lacking social support, fractured community and family structures, growing inequality, fewer pro-social behaviours, and unchanged levels of average life satisfaction (Hossain et al., 2007; Pretty et al., 2015). Some of these find expression in the fast-increasing incidence of obesity, type 2 diabetes, mental ill-health, dementias, some cancers, and cardiovascular disease (Hossain et al., 2007). Mental disorders now account for a large proportion of the disease burden in many countries, affecting 13–20 per cent of 12–24 year olds in most industrialised countries (Patel et al., 2007), though it is important to note that perceptions of what constitutes mental ill-health have changed over the decades

(Phelan et al., 2000). Communities and indeed whole countries have become wealthier, yet increased material consumption has displaced important protective life choices and behaviours that are in turn partly conditioned by policy and markets (Layard, 2006; Royal Society, 2012).

It is now clear that continuing increases in GDP in affluent countries have not been associated with increases in well-being (Royal Society, 2012; Pretty, 2013). Latitudinal analyses across countries show a characteristic consumption cliff and affluent uplands shape: at low per capita GDP, well-being increases with rising GDP; after a threshold, well-being is largely independent of GDP across the affluent uplands (Figure 1.1). More surprisingly, longitudinal analyses over 50–60 years show that well-being in already affluent countries has remained resolutely stable even though per capita GDP has risen (e.g. between 3 and 8 fold in the UK, USA and Japan) (Figure 1.2).

Despite the apparent lack of well-being dividend once countries have become affluent by GDP or other consumption measures, consumption patterns in many countries continue to converge on those of the richest. As the poorer take similar choices, seeking to use natural capital and environmental services in similarly damaging ways, so pressure on both natural and social systems grows (MEA, 2005; NEA, 2011).

Previous research has shown that the factors of consumption between different country groups are still substantially different (Table 1.1). Vehicle ownership in the Affluent North America-Europe-Oceania countries is 91 times greater than in the poorest countries, and in Affluent Asia 54 times greater than the poorest. Oil

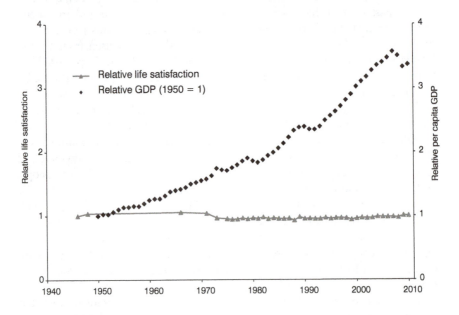

Figure 1.1 Changes in per capita GDP and life satisfaction, UK (1946–2011) (Pretty, 2013)

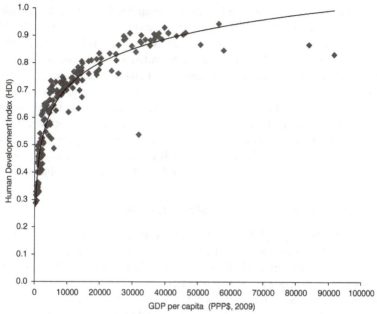

Figure 1.2 Relationship between GDP and HDI at country level (n=173) (Pretty, 2013)

Table 1.1 Factors of consumption from poorest to fast developing and most affluent countries

Consumption metrics	Poorest to Affluent North America–Europe–Oceania	Poorest to Affluent Asia	Fast developing (BRICs and CIVETS) to Affluent North America–Europe–Oceania	Fast developing (BRICs and CIVETS) to Affluent Asia
Motor vehicles	91.4×	54.3×	5.3×	3.2×
Domestic water	28.5×	16.6×	2.3×	1.4×
CO$_2$ emissions	118.0×	90.0×	2.7×	2.1×
Oil consumption	38.0×	97.3×	3.9×	10.0×
Meat consumption	11.9×	4.8×	2.3×	1.3×

Note: BRICs are Brazil, Russia, India, China; CIVETS are Colombia, Indonesia, Vietnam, Turkey and South Africa

Source: Pretty (2013)

consumption in the Affluent North America-Europe-Oceania countries is four times greater than in the fastest developing countries. With world population expected to rise by 2–3 billion from the current 7.5 billion by mid-century before stabilising (assuming low- to medium-fertility scenarios), this will add further to consumption.

The global metrics developed to demonstrate the impacts of human activities on finite Earth conclude that at current world population and existing levels of consumption, planetary overshoot has already occurred. These include the Human Development Index (UNDP), Genuine Progress Indicator (Daly and Cobb, 1989), Ecological Footprints using global hectare equivalents (WWF, 2012), the Happy Planet Index (NEF, 2013), and planetary boundaries (Rockstrom et al., 2009). Overshoot implies more resources are being used than can be regenerated each year. Climate change is likely to be one of the indicators of the negative side-effects of such consumption (IPCC, 2013). The Royal Society (2012) stated that indefinite growth is impossible in a finite world, yet conventional economic growth remains a primary goal in most countries. As a result, behaviours and policy choices that improve well-being and health tend to have been displaced, despite the fact that GDP continues to be used as a poor proxy for sustainable and equitable prosperity.

Tackling well-being and health challenges

The term 'health' is generally taken to incorporate physical health, mental or emotional health, social health, spiritual health, lifestyle and functionality. The World Health Organization (1948) definition of health remains the most widely cited and states that "health is a state of complete physical, mental and social (individual) well-being, and not merely the absence of disease or infirmity". In a similar way, well-being is a positive physical, social and mental state; it is not just the absence of pain, discomfort and incapacity. It requires that basic needs are met, that individuals have a sense of purpose, that they feel able to achieve important personal goals and participate in society (Pencheon, 2012; ONS, 2013).

It is unlikely that apparently wealthy countries will have the financial capability to spend the necessary additional resources to solve the next wave of health problems brought about by high material consumption, unless new models of health and social care are developed. Jackson (2009) concluded that modern society has been "betrayed by affluence", and Dasgupta (2010) observed that "the rogue word in GDP is gross", as it does not deduct the costly depreciation of vital natural and social assets. A concept of the wealth of nations should include measures for natural capital, social capital and individual well-being. GDP currently does not (Pretty, 2013). This suggests the need to prioritise new interventions to improve well-being and health and combine these with existing medical treatments. Such interventions should focus on both direct treatment of individuals and the contextual conditioning brought about by social and natural environments. These external environments condition internal physiological, hormonal and neural pathways, which in turn directly influence well-being and health. In this way, health is no longer described as simply a lack of disease, and highlights the need to revisit our (often contextual) framing of what it means to be healthy.

In the past two decades, a wide range of empirical evidence has emerged to show that well-being is improved by physical activity, diet and nutrition, direct engagement with nature and green places, attachments to people, attachments to personal possessions, the mind, and the fulfilment of values. The evidence has implications for the design of health and social care systems (models of care, hospitals and other health and care service buildings), transport policy, green space availability and use, food systems, social care policy and practice, the work place, leisure choices and child policy.

Evidence further suggests that there are substantial economic, financial and environmental gains to be made by adopting new interventions and choices (CMO, 2013). There remains, however, some scepticism and misunderstanding over both the evidence and its potentially powerful implications. Evidence to support seven interconnected themes of Asclepian healing is increasingly challenging some of the tenets of modern health care, the most powerful of which is that not all health care currently does good, and that much health care is important and needed largely because we have failed to create societies, cultures and economies that promote well-being.

Heresy 1: Sensory inputs from natural places improve well-being

The natural environment provides important ecosystem services that underpin economies (MEA, 2005; NEA, 2011). It also provides health services (Pretty et al., 2011; Jackson et al., 2013). Ecosystems provide four generic health benefits i) direct positive effects on mental and physical health; ii) indirect positive effects by facilitating nature-based activity and social engagement (providing locations for contact with nature, physical activity and social engagement), all of which positively influence health, and catalysing behavioural change towards healthier lifestyles (improving life pathways, activity behaviour, consumption of healthy foods); iii) reducing the threats to health arising from pollution and disease vectors (through purification and control functions, such as local climate regulation, noise reduction, and scavenging of air pollutants), and iv) direct benefits to health care: e.g. most drugs can trace their origin back to natural products (from simple painkillers to complex anti-cancer drugs); and there are likely to be many more undiscovered therapies if we appreciate the important role of millions of years of evolution (e.g. through biomimicry).

Detailed scientific evidence has confirmed there are direct health benefits of light, colour, whole views, bird song and scents (Pretty et al., 2005; Joye et al., 2013; Ratcliffe et al., 2013). The view from the window enhances well-being and healing in hospitals and prisons (Moore, 1982; Ulrich, 1984), and views with natural elements (e.g. trees, green space, blue sky and water) have a positive effect while those with urban structures have a negative effect. Nature-dominated drives increase recovery from stress: commuters recover quicker from stress and reduce the likelihood of future stresses after nature-drives compared with urban-dominated drives. Urban areas with plentiful tree cover and green space have been shown to have children with a lower prevalence of asthma (though this may be because certain kinds of social groups are able to live in these areas), improved mental well-being, reductions in stress, positive effects on birth outcomes, lower morbidity, reduced cardiovascular disease (CVD) risk, greater longevity of the elderly and positive effects on cognitive function (Takano et al., 2002; Hartig, 2008; Lovasi et al., 2008; Mitchell and Popham, 2008; Park et al., 2008; Maas et al., 2009; Barton and Pretty, 2010; Bratman et al., 2012; Dadvand et al., 2012). More green space results in healthier cortisol profiles; less green space typical of deprived communities produce higher stress and flattened cortisol profiles (indicating poorer capacity to recover from stress) and increased incidence of obesity (Lachowycz and Jones, 2011; Roe et al., 2013).

Further direct benefits arise from sunlight, which is important for vitamin D manufacture in the body, thus having a direct impact on health. Ultra violet B is absorbed by dehydrocholesterol in the skin, which is further converted to vitamin D3, and metabolised by the liver to a biologically active form. Lack of vitamin D causes rickets in children, cases of which in the UK rose from 147 in 1997 to 762 in 2010, as well as exacerbating osteoporosis and osteomalacia in adults. More recently it has been recognised that vitamin D deficiency is associated with increased risks of some cancers, CVD, multiple sclerosis, rheumatoid arthritis, and type 1 diabetes, with possible links to type 2 diabetes and schizophrenia, even though increased skin cancer incidence is related to too much exposure to sunlight (Kampman et al., 2007; Perrine et al., 2010; Juniper, 2013).

Heresy 2: Regular physical activity improves both mental and physical health

It is well-known that physical activity improves both mental and physical health (CDC, 1996; Foresight, 2007; DoH, 2009). Physical inactivity results in 1.9 million deaths worldwide annually, roughly 1 in 25 of all deaths. Energy expenditure has fallen dramatically over the past half-century; pre-industrial people typically expended 1000 kcal on activity per day, whereas for moderns the average is only 300 kcal (Samson and Pretty, 2006). Inactivity increases the likelihood of obesity, and reduces life expectancy. Such physical inactivity is known to track from childhood, and is a key risk factor in many chronic diseases of later life (Wichstrom et al., 2013).

The costs of inactivity in the UK exceed £8.3 billion per year (NICE, 2009). In the UK alone, some 23 per cent of men and 26 per cent of women are sedentary. A 1 per cent reduction in inactivity (or a 1 per cent increase in activity), reduces morbidity by 15,000 cases and saves £1.4 billion. Never in human history have humans, as a species, moved bodies so far with so little physical effort. The benefits amount to £2420 per additionally active person per year (not including the mental health benefits). In the USA, sedentary behaviour costs $90 billion per year, and it is estimated that some 30,000 deaths could be prevented with adoption of regular physical activity (Brownson et al., 2005).

Ekblom-Bak et al. (2013) have coined the term *non-exercise physical activity* (NEPA) to draw attention to the health benefits of daily activities such as home repairs, cutting the lawn, car maintenance, bicycle rides, fishing and gathering mushrooms and berries: 60-year old Swedish men and women with high NEPA reduced the risk of first time CVD by 27 per cent and all-cause mortality by 30 per cent over a 12.5-year period. The term *green exercise* was coined to indicate the potentially synergistic well-being benefits arising from activity in green places (Pretty et al., 2005; Barton et al., 2009). A dose of nature (Barton and Pretty, 2010) has been shown to have an immediate positive effect on mental health for a wide range of activities (e.g. walking, angling, cycling, gardening), for all age groups, for men and women, for every green environment and habitat (with additional benefits from the presence of water), and for the already healthy and the mentally ill. Forest bathing (walking) in Japan reduces blood pressure and salivary cortisol, with greater benefits shown for the elderly and those already with high blood pressure and more stress markers (Li, this volume, pp. 79-88).

Green care arises from green exercise, and is the deliberate use of structured therapeutic programmes using walking, gardening and/or farming (Sempik and Bragg, this volume, pp. 100–113). It has been successfully applied for youth offenders, the self-declared mentally ill (e.g. *Mind* members), those suffering from dementias and post-traumatic stress (Mapes, this volume, pp. 150–160). In this way, attentiveness and mindfulness, outdoor activities and well-being can all be linked (Christie, 2013).

Heresy 3: The mind alone can improve well-being

The notion of the separate entities of mind and body has become outdated, as it is now clear that thought alone can cascade physiological pathways that influence well-being. There are two important evidence bases: from research on contemplation arising from mindfulness and prayer, and from research on the placebo effect.

Many philosophical, spiritual and psychological traditions emphasise the importance of the quality of consciousness on well-being. Mindfulness emphasises attentiveness to the present reality, with focused awareness providing heightened sensitivity, and is defined as paying attention in a particular way; on purpose, in the present moment and non-judgementally (Williams and Penman, 2011). It can be contrasted with states of mind in which attention is focused elsewhere, including preoccupation with plans or worries, and behaving automatically without paying attention to your actions. Such attentiveness may be external or internal, such as on breathing patterns. Mindfulness can be cultivated by practice, and has led to therapeutic uses through Mindfulness-Based Stress Reduction (MBSR) which has been effective with patients with anxiety or persistent pain (Nyklíček and Kuijpers, 2008; Shapiro et al., 2008; Williams and Penman, 2011). In some contexts, mindfulness is used as a means to develop compassion for self and others, leading to observed reductions in stress and increases in quality of life. It has also been shown to increase enzyme activity that builds up telomeres, thus extending longevity (Jacobs et al., 2011).

A similar literature exists for prayer: the sending of prayer has no effect if the recipient does not know it is being practised; for those undertaking prayer it improves well-being (Dusek et al., 2002; Benson et al., 2006). Frequency of prayer and prayer experiences is a good predictor of well-being (Poloma and Pendleton, 1991), though this may be association rather than causation. The combination of mindfulness and exercise, such as by practising tai chi, improves well-being and produces stronger immune responses in practitioners. Lutz et al. (2008) showed that meditation cultivates positive emotions, and these alter brain circuitry linked to empathy, and relaxation through meditation, prayer, yoga and tai chi are all associated with instant decreased oxygen consumption, reduced blood pressure and heart rate, and increased serotonin and dopamine levels (Esch et al., 2003). Being in natural places further encourages attentiveness in many people, though it is not clear whether natural spaces support the ability to be mindful, or whether practitioners of mindfulness experience more positive health benefits when spending time in nature.

Yet something uncomfortable must also be concluded for this rational age: the decline of spirituality and attendance at formal religious ceremonies has removed some opportunities for engagement with community and place, and may have influenced well-being as well as negatively influenced the capability to cope with stress (Koenig, 2000). Modern society has become indifferent to, or even discouraging of, spiritual traditions, especially in the public sphere (Walker, 2011). Material culture has tended to fill the gap.

Recent research on the placebo effect (PE) has further shown the potential benefits of "self-healing". The placebo has long been conceptualised as an inert process, and thus has been used both as a control in experiments and to separate imagination from reality. It is now known to be a genuine phenomenon, with thought leading to expectancy to effect (Finniss et al., 2010). Expectancy is critical, and beliefs and expectations are important in both patient and physicians/nurses. The PE has yielded beneficial clinical results for angina, bronchial asthma, herpes, ulcers, inflammatory bowel syndrome, and persistent pain (Enck et al., 2008; Kaptchuk et al., 2008; Price et al., 2008; Zubieta and Stohler, 2009). The largest amount of research has been on analgesics, which has shown that the PE mechanism centres on the self-release of endogenous opioids. The PE has been shown to be blocked if opioid inhibitors, such as naloxone, are given to patients. Fuente-Fernandez et al. (2001) used PET scanning to show that Parkinson's disease patients substantially increase dopamine releases in response to placebos, and concluded that PE can be a powerful treatment.

The "open–hidden" paradigm is important: hidden treatment is generally ineffective, thus both patient and physician must expect a treatment to work. Finniss et al. (2010) noted that effective alternative therapies with no clear scientific explanation but with elaborate rituals can thus induce placebo effects, particularly if there is a good relationship between practitioner and patient. PE is also accompanied by reduced neural activity in brain areas that process pain and anxiety. Kaptchuk et al. (2008) concluded that "augmented treatment" with warmth, attention, and confidence improves clinical outcomes. Patients thus engage in treating themselves if physicians, nurses and carers have a warm friendly manner, engage in active listening, show empathy, allow up to 20 seconds of silence in conversation, and communicate confidence and positive expectations. Compassion is important to recovery, and is clearly a crucial part of the whole patient experience, one of the three dimensions of quality in the English national health system, alongside safety and effectiveness.

There remain important ethical issues over patient deception with respect to PE and self-healing, though Kaptchuk et al. (2010) have shown how placebos without deception can work in trials to treat irritable bowel syndrome. One conclusion from the placebo research is that there exists some capacity to improve well-being without the need for drug interventions.

Heresy 4: The immune system can be trained to work better, especially from childhood

Recent research has demonstrated that social and environmental context and individual behaviour choices have a long-term effect on well-being and health. Multi-decade longitudinal cohort studies indicate clearly that many of the social and environmental conditions of childhood can predict adult health status. These include the 1972 Dunedin (now 40+ years after start), Cambridge (48 years after), Maudsley (21 years) and the Whitehall studies (Danner et al., 2001; Marmot and Bruner, 2004; Foresight, 2008). Danner et al. (2001) investigated the autobiographies that a group of ageing nuns had written six decades earlier at the age of about 20. Since then, their ways of living had been very similar, yet those in the lower half of the cohort when ranked for positive comments about life died nine years earlier than those in the top half. Positive mental health affected survival 60 years later in life.

It is clear that there is considerable tracking from childhood to adulthood. Ill-health tracks, and childhood mental ill-health is especially carried forward (Foresight, 2008). It has been shown that 80 per cent of children of low socioeconomic status become overweight adults, whereas only 40 per cent of those with high status become overweight (Wells and Lekies, 2006). Such tracking, though, is clearer from adolescence than early childhood. Early socially-stimulating environments are, however, crucial, with later emotional well-being and cognitive capacity profoundly influenced by early social development (Ainsworth et al., 1974).

This suggests a need to establish good behaviours early (Louv, 2005). Engagement with wild nature secures positive adult outcomes, and a visit to woodland as a child increases the number of visits made as an adult (Ward Thompson et al., 2008). Play affects brain development. Outdoor activity has a positive effect on long-term memory, and cognitive development is influenced by free play and exploration (Rickinson et al., 2004; Berman et al., 2008).

Related to the placebo effect is the concept of conditioning, the training of the body to react in a particular way to stimuli. Both expectancy and memory can be important. The repeated association between a neural stimulus and an active drug can result in the ability of the neural stimulus to elicit a response on its own (Finniss et al., 2010). Ader and Cohen (2002) showed that in subjects repeatedly given cyclosporin and a flavoured drink, immunosuppression was induced. At a later point, the same subjects given only the flavoured drink again responded with induced immunosuppression. Other subjects with no prior conditioning showed no suppression when given only the flavoured drink. Memory is important, as recollection of a previous placebo magnitude influences future treatment effects. In this way, once again, drug-like effects can be induced without drugs (Enck et al., 2008).

Heresy 5: Social bonds and attachment between people improves well-being

Insel and Young (2001) have written: "it is difficult to think of any behavioural process that is more important to us than attachment". Attachment behaviour has emerged in humans as there are selective advantages to enduring bonds. The neuropeptide, oxytocin, has been shown to be a critical compound, and oxytocin receptors are concentrated in the dopamine-rich regions of the brain. Oxytocin can be released by touching, by being in safe environments, and on receiving signals of trust from others. Those with high levels of oxytocin or high numbers of receptors have a greater ability to empathise and increased motivations to be generous. Zak et al. (2007) have shown that subjects given oxytocin become more generous. Those who volunteer to help others are known also to have higher well-being (McCloughlan et al., 2011). Across the EU, 20 per cent of citizens participate in volunteering and charitable activities, the highest proportions are in Denmark, Finland and Sweden (>45 per cent). Volunteering is associated with improved happiness, self-esteem, sense of control and wider mental health; those attending religious ceremonies are more likely to volunteer (Thoits and Hewitt, 2001; Mellor, 2009; McCloughlan et al., 2011). In this way, the seven heresies are interlinked.

It is well-established that trusting relationships have an effect on health (Kawachi et al., 1997). Conversely isolation and negative feelings affect health negatively (Ostrom, 1990). The value attached to relationships constitutes a form of capital, which has come to be known as social capital. This includes an individual's contacts and networks; the common rules, norms and sanctions that regulate behaviour together with the reciprocity and exchanges that build friendships, respect and ultimately trust (Pretty and Ward, 2001).

Three types of social capital are commonly identified. These are i) bonding: the ability to engage positively with those closest who share similar values; ii) bridging: working effectively with those who have dissimilar values and goals; and iii) linking: the ability to engage positively with those in authority either to influence their policies or obtain resources (Pretty, 2003). A central theme of Putnam's bowling alone thesis (1995) was that although just as many people in the USA participate in ten-pin bowling as they did half a century earlier, they tended now to bowl alone or in small groups of existing friends. When individuals were members of competitive teams in a league, then they played teams from other social and ethnic groups within cities, and as a result bridging social capital was built through regular contact. Such social attachment increases well-being (Esch and Stefano, 2005); mothers with strong attachment to their infants show greater activation of brain reward regions, especially of the oxytocin-associated hypothalamus, but insecure mothers showed much reduced responses.

It is clear that people engage with the outdoors not just for the connection to nature, but to provide the setting for the building of social capital. Nature is good for health; green places are good for social capital. Strong social support keeps the elderly alive, and membership of sports clubs contributes to well-being. A meta-analysis of 148 studies (Holt-Lunstad et al., 2010) found a 50 per cent increased likelihood of survival over seven years for those people with strong relationships.

The opposite of social attachment is loneliness. This has a directly negative effect on health, and thus a reduction in loneliness will improve well-being. The study of loneliness has demonstrated the biological effect of a lack of social relationships (Miller, 2011). Lonely adults tend to have higher blood pressure, greater epinephrine secretion at night, higher morning and night-time cortisol levels, and poorer sleep patterns (Glaser et al., 1985; Hawkley and Cacioppo, 2007). Short visits by carers may not help, as the quality of friendships and compassionate time spent together is important. The chronic stress experienced by carers themselves reduces immune responses to vaccines and slows wound healing (Kiecolt-Glaser et al., 1996). Stress plays a major role in neurodegenerative disease, mental disorder and memory. Both cortisol and epinephrine are markers of stress, and people who lack social support are more prone to ailments and illness (Hawkley and Cacioppo, 2007). Cortisol plays a key role in the HPA (hypothalmic-pituitary-adrenocortical) axis, which controls inflammatory processes and maintains immune function. Loneliness increases gene activity that promotes inflammation, and with poorer sleep and reduced night-time repair, ill-health outcomes increase. Loneliness tracks into adulthood, with lonely adults having a greater number of childhood adversities such as hospitalisation, parental divorce and physical abuse (Asher and Paquette, 2003; Hawkley and Cacioppo, 2007).

In the USA, 29 million people live alone, a 30 per cent increase since 1980, and people are three times more likely now to report having no one to talk to. Social exclusion decreases prosocial behaviour, and is related to higher anxiety, increased loneliness and more mental ill-health (Twenge et al., 2007), though higher social class is often associated with less prosocial behaviour (Piff et al., 2012). In the UK, 10 per cent of over 65-year-olds are always or very lonely (900,000 people), and half of all 75-year-olds live alone (Campaign to End Loneliness, 2015). Loneliness has the equivalent risk as consuming 15 cigarettes per day and is twice as harmful as obesity (Bolton, 2012). Lonely people make more visits to GPs and attend A&E more often. Befriending, mentoring, wayfinding and gatekeeper services and group activities such as walking for health, have been shown to reduce hospital and health care costs. After such interventions, mean visits to GPs fall from 10.8 to 6.7 per year (Pitkala et al., 2009). Attachment and oxytocin interact to suppress anxiety and physiological stress (Tops et al., 2007). This suggests the need for access to green space for all social groups, and a role for green space in cities to play in reducing health inequalities (Kuo and Sullivan, 2001; Marmot Review, 2008).

Heresy 6: Attachment to possessions and place with emotional history improves well-being

Consumer culture has increased the turnover of possessions, and may also have undermined self and identity, thus also reducing well-being (Tuan, 1977; Belk, 1988; Walker, 2011). Sartre noted that people seek, express and confirm a sense of being through their possessions, and Marx used the term "commodity fetishism" to indicate the structural relations of capitalism that result in detachment, with consumers coming to believe commodities have some kind of power to make them happy (Jackson, 2006). Yet Walker (2011) has observed that "our contemporary market system sells, more than anything else, discontent and unhappiness". The modern economy needs disposal and replacement; it is centred on ephemerality. Yet if people become more attached to both possessions and natural places, and thus do not purchase new goods or repair harm to ecosystems, then the economy will suffer (unless a different kind of prosperity based on well-being is pursued: Pretty, 2013). In contradiction, the planet would benefit incrementally from each increase in attachment. When possessions and places acquire a high degree of attachment for people, then they are less likely to be disposed of or damaged. Importantly, high attachment and affiliation also improve mental and physical well-being.

Cathexis is the process of charging an object, activity or place with emotional energy (Belk, 1988), which in turn emerges from memory creation. Attachments are formed with specific material objects, evolve over time, emerge from experience and personal history, and are thus a form of self-expression (Schultz et al., 1989; Belk, 1991). Cherished possessions with such meaning tend not to be substituted and, therefore, are more likely to be kept for a long time, becoming inalienable wealth or capital for families (Bell, 1997; Curasi et al., 2005). This in turn leads to greater well-being: cherished possessions and places with high affiliation value result in higher life satisfaction and well-being (Sherman and Newman, 1977). This has been recognised in hospitals and care-settings: patients and the elderly are viewed as more socially-capable and less dependent by medical and care staff if they display personal possessions in wards and rooms (Millard and Smith, 1981; Wapner et al., 1990). People with possessions are more in control, less helpless, and more supported by staff. Recovering heart surgery patients with views of trees are more likely to have positive comments written about them by hospital staff (Ulrich, 2002).

People also invest more in possessions and natural capital when either or both are cathected and charged with emotional energy. The more strongly homeowners cathect their dwellings, for example, the more frequently they invest in mowing grass, painting, cleaning and remodelling. Sherman and Newman (1977) showed that the elderly with family possessions depicting grandchildren and key events, relationships and memories are happier than those who do not. When people are deprived of their valued possessions and places, their personal identity is harmed too (Albrecht, 2005). Possessions linked to memorable past events help to verify that the event occurred, and emotions (good and bad) are fixers of memory. In this way, possessions and green places can be thought of as magical vessels, carrying the power of kratophany and expressing stories, values and memories that are tangible proof of life events (Belk, 1991; Curasi et al., 2005; Kane, 2010; Christie, 2013).

Heresy 7: The design within buildings and settlements influences well-being

Design within buildings and settlements influences well-being, today usually for the worse. Buildings and settlements are part-planned in advance, and part emergent and changed according to contemporary needs (Brand, 1994; Orr, 2006; Walker, 2011). In the modern era, buildings tend no longer to care for users' and visitors' well-being, and sadly not even for staff; and settlements discourage activities and behaviours that would improve well-being, forcing people into care, reducing social interaction, and reducing time spent in nature. The hospice movement has long-understood the need to create a therapeutic health care environment, but hospitals have not (BMA, 2011). The hospital environment plays a significant role in staff and patient functioning, yet largely they are noisy, devoid of natural views or internal plants, do not use natural light or sunlight effectively, and do not provide places where visitors and/or staff can socially-interact. Ulrich (2002) concluded that many hospitals are "starkly stressful, unacceptably stressful, and unsuited to the emotional needs of patients, their families and even health care staff". Becoming ill is a stressful experience, and design makes this worse (Kings Fund, 2009; BMA, 2011).

The typically high levels of boredom and few opportunities for physical activity further undermine recovery. There is a tendency to focus much energy on how good or bad structures are, but relatively little attention is paid to the overall health and care system. Better models of prevention and care should be the priority and the structures needed to support such a system. This suggests more transformational models are needed. The built environment and the shared, open, natural environment have important negative and positive direct consequences on health and are powerful influences on health-related behaviours. In particular, future-proofed environments need to be flexible (easy to change function), adaptable (easy to refurbish) and aesthetic (the health care environment has a particular responsibility to be both health-promoting and therapeutic).

Patients in east-facing rooms exposed to more light from early in the day spend less time on the ward and have lower mortality (Even et al., 2008). Private, allotment and community gardens have all been shown to reduce stress and improve well-being, as has green space in deprived communities (Ward Thompson et al., 2012; Hawkins et al., 2013; Twiss et al., 2013). Having your own garden has also been shown to be restorative, again reducing stress. School gardens are important for pupil behaviour as well as outdoor learning (Ofsted, 2008).

Gardens in hospitals also have a number of positive effects on individuals, by helping them to feel more relaxed and able to cope, reducing stress and improving mood (Cooper-Marcus and Barnes, 1999). Even short visits to gardens of five minutes in duration have been demonstrated to have a positive effect on the mental well-being of patients (Barton and Pretty, 2010). Loud noise, though, increases stress, raises blood pressure and heart rates: noise is a major cause of sleep deprivation in hospitals, yet sleep is necessary for vital immune and endocrine functions (BMA, 2011). The TLC (Turning off unused equipment, switching off Lights, and Closing hospital doors) programme at Barts Health NHS Trust has already saved substantial sums of money through behaviour change (Barts Health NHS Trust, 2013).

Design thus matters. The Royal Children's Hospital in Melbourne integrates nature into the hospital by replaced facades, creating virtual and digital landscapes, has a seven metre aquarium in the waiting area, and has windows, skylights and viewing platforms to bring the neighbouring park into the building (Green, 2013). The BMA (2011) concluded that a therapeutic health care environment would induce positive clinical outcomes, reduce drug consumption, shorten average lengths of stay, create better doctor–patient relationships, and improve mental well-being. The social climate in hospitals should promote vital social bonds, which in turn improve well-being.

Saving money and increasing well-being

A largely unchallenged assumption for the past half century has been that increased material consumption and rising GDP leads to increased well-being. Now a priority is to redefine prosperity, and by substituting activities that improve social cohesion, happiness, mental and physical well-being, and memory creation for material consumption, the impact on natural capital and ecosystem services will be reduced whilst improving well-being. Green growth and the green economy have become important targets for national and international organisations (Boyle and Simms, 2009; O'Neill et al., 2010; Pretty, 2013). UNEP (2011) defines the green economy as "resulting in human well-being and social equity, while significantly reducing environmental risks and ecological scarcities".

A green-health economy that emphasises ecological public health would be one in which attention is paid to the environmental and social context of the public not yet ill, patients and all professionals and families engaged in treatment and care (Pencheon, 2012; CMO, 2013). The Marmot Review (2008) of health inequalities concluded that "economic growth is not the most important measure of our country's success", and recommended attention to accumulate the positive effects on well-being across the whole life course by building social capital, encouraging active travel, use of public transport, availability of green space and healthy eating. A particular concern centres on the sometimes sharp social gradients of health: childhood mortality in regions of the UK varies from 7 to 23/100,000; mental ill-health in children comprises 17 per cent of those in families with no educational qualifications yet only 4 per cent of those with degrees (CMO, 2013).

The UK Office for National Statistics is now measuring well-being at the national level in the UK; but these measures have largely not changed policy or practice, particularly in health and social care. Hospitals have evolved considerably since their first establishment in Mesopotamia 3000 years ago (Retief and Ciliers, 2006), yet health and social care now needs to enter another phase of development. Mitchell and Popham (2008) concluded that "environments that promote good health might be crucial in the fight to reduce health inequalities". The role of organised societal efforts can be to remove barriers and simply to create the right conditions for social resilience and health to develop naturally in communities.

Asclepian temples engaged in healing by combining the use of drugs obtained from medicinal plants alongside lengthy stays in temple surroundings, the use of dream rooms, hydrotherapy, exercise, healthy foods and the library. The caduceul staff of Asclepius depicts the harmless temple serpent, *Zamenis longissimus*, coiled around the staff, the snake a symbol of rejuvenation for its shedding of skin and ability to assume the shape of a circle, a symbol of eternity. It also kept temples free of rats, and came to represent a pluralistic approach to medical healing and treatment (Hart, 1965; Oberhelman, 2013). An Asclepian staff and snake is carved onto a relief at Sulis Minerva, one of the baths built by the Romans at Bath and used for some two centuries as a location for healing.

A substantial financial dividend would be released by a green-health economy centred on interconnected Asclepian principles of healing and well-being:

i.   regular engagement with nature;
ii.   regular physical activity (alongside healthy and available food);
iii. use of the power of thought and contemplation;
iv.   train the immune system from childhood;
v.   enhance social bonds;
vi.   increase attachment to possessions and places;
vii. redesign buildings and settlements, and create shared space, to ensure interaction and attachment.

This suggests there would be co-benefits from consideration of amended models of health care delivery, in which the primary location of care is the home and community setting, and the most appropriate need is translated into demand for general practitioner surgeries, leaving hospitals to focus on specialist care that cannot be delivered closer to home. This would be good for the health of patients, the public, the national economy and state of the planet: an important and wide range of co-benefits. Every unplanned admission is in some ways a sign of system failure. Health and care services must thus become more imaginative, flexible and human. In doing so, they would also become more financially viable and efficient. This will in turn need to create business models for sustainable health and social care that focus more on incentivising prevention and outcomes rather than simply rewarding activity.

It is clear that environmental and social context influences well-being and health, and thus actions that shape these contexts for individuals will increase the likelihood that more people will be able to live their lives well and for longer, as well as leave a better legacy for all.

Chapter 2

Nature in buildings and health design

Stephen R. Kellert

Biophilia and biophilic design

Theory backed by a growing body of evidence increasingly indicates people possess an inherent inclination to affiliate with the non-human environment – other species and the natural habitats, systems, and processes we commonly refer to as nature (Kellert 2012). This theory has been called Biophilia (Wilson 1986, Kellert and Wilson 1993, Kellert 1997, 2012). Biophilia represents an understanding of human evolutionary biology, recognizing that for almost all human history our species evolved in adaptive response to largely natural not artificial forces and stimuli. Indeed, much of what we regard as 'normal' today is of relatively recent origin – the invention of large-scale agriculture some 10–12,000 years ago, the creation of the city some 5–6000 years ago, industrial revolution 2–300 years ago, and lately the electronic era. As a consequence, the human body, mind, and senses evolutionarily developed under mainly the pressure of bio-centric not human invented or engineered factors.

The result is that we are biologically programmed to respond to a wide variety of environmental cues and natural stimuli. A classic study by the Swedish psychologist, Arne Öhman (1986, Ulrich 1993), found that people subliminally exposed to pictures of snakes, spiders, frayed electric wires, and handguns, elicited largely aversive reactions to snakes and spiders and indifference to the more modern threats. This study is both illustrative and cautionary. It demonstrates the continued emotive power of features and forces of the natural environment, but also that at least some of these reactions can be viewed as vestigial, reactions that evolved under once adaptive circumstances, but that today have become largely irrelevant and will likely eventually atrophy over time.

Despite this possibility, a growing body of empirical data increasingly suggests many of our inherent affinities for the natural world continue to be instrumental in human physical and mental health and well-being. While the evidence supporting this relationship is not extensive and the studies often methodologically limited, the breadth of the findings across a wide variety of disciplines and human endeavours cumulatively supports the impression that certain forms of contact with nature remain important in human health, fitness and well-being. This relationship has been revealed in studies of nature contact in educational, office, manufacturing, residential, community, and healthcare settings (Kellert 2012).

In the healthcare field, studies have reported exposure to nature can result in stress relief, muscle relaxation, lower blood pressure, reduced cortisol levels, mitigation of pain, and healing and illness recovery (Searles 1960, Friedmann 1983, Katcher 1993, Ulrich 1993, Frumkin 2001, Taylor 2001, Frumkin 2008, Kellert and Heerwagen 2008, Ulrich 2008, Cama 2009, Bowler et al., 2010, 2008, Kuo 2010, Townsend and Weerasuriya 2010, Annerstedt and Währborg 2011, Kellert 2012, Louv 2012, Wells and Rollings 2012, Marcus and Sachs 2014). In addition, other research and anecdotal evidence indicates contact with nature can have significant healthcare operational benefits including increased comfort, satisfaction, motivation, morale, and performance of hospital staff, improved employee recruitment and retention, and reduced conflicts among patients, staff, and hospital visitors (Ulrich 2008, Kellert and Finnegan 2011).

Despite the apparent continuing importance of contact with nature, a number of obstacles exist in modern society to the adaptive and robust occurrence of biophilia. Of particular importance, biophilia is a weak not hard-wired biological tendency, which like much of what makes us human is heavily reliant on learning, experience, and social support to develop fully and functionally (Wilson 1986, Kellert 2012). This dependence on learning is what allows humanity to be inventive and distinctive as individuals and societies, but also permits people by equal measure to behave in self-destructive and self-defeating ways. With respect to biophilia, people can either engage the natural world in an adaptive or, conversely, inadequate and counter-productive manner. Unfortunately, for various historical and cultural reasons (Kellert 2012), modern society has increasingly separated itself from the ongoing experience of nature, having largely concluded the natural world is just raw material to be converted through human inventiveness to higher and better uses or a nice but not necessary recreational amenity. This assumption is reflected in modern agriculture, manufacturing, architecture, urbanization, healthcare, and elsewhere.

In modern healthcare, the prevailing medical model views illness as largely a physical malady to be remedied through technical means. Reflecting this bias, healthcare facilities are usually highly antiseptic and technologically dominated environments, which routinely exclude non-human nature as either irrelevant or a potential threat. As a consequence, the typical healthcare facility is a featureless, sensory-deprived setting devoid of natural forms and features.

The design of the built environment is especially critical in modern society as the natural habitat of contemporary humans has mainly become a constructed world. Our species may have evolved in nature, but today we spend most of our time indoors in a human created and designed setting. Moreover, some four-fifths of the population in industrially-developed countries now live in an urban area, historically the most environmentally transformed, degraded, and artificial of all human habitats, where people routinely separate themselves from ongoing contact with nature. This contemporary shift away from the natural world has been exacerbated by the exponential growth of electronic technology. Recent data reveals the typical American child is engaged with electronic media more than fifty hours each week, while outside involved in free play less than one hour during a typical day (Kaiser Family Foundation 2005, Louv 2005).

Before concluding modern humans have become largely disconnected from the natural world, it is important to recognize the experience of nature can occur in multiple ways. The most obvious form is direct contact with the natural world in outdoor settings. In addition, people experience 'indirect' contact with nature through various interactions that involve continuous human input and control such as a potted plant, a garden, aquarium, pet animals, and more. Finally, people experience nature vicariously and representationally through pictures, symbols, stories, recordings, television, video, computers, and more. All forms of contact with the natural world – direct, indirect and representational – are important to human health and well-being, although no effective substitute exists for the unparalleled benefits of direct experience as a consequence of its multisensory, dynamic, continuously changing, unpredictable, and ambient qualities (Sebba 1991, Pyle 1993, Kellert 2012).

Biophilic design of healthcare facilities

Assuming the validity of the biophilia hypothesis that people continue to rely on contact with nature for health and well-being, a fundamental challenge is how to ensure this occurs in the modern built environment. Given the prevalence of the built environment in modern life, this challenge is one of what has been called biophilic design: the design of buildings and constructed landscapes that foster human health and well-being through contact with nature in constructed settings of cultural and ecological significance (Kellert et al., 2008, Kellert and Finnegan 2011).

The basic objective of biophilic design is to create good habitat for people as a biological organism in the built environment. A number of principles derive from this understanding, biophilic design should:

1 focus on human adaptations to the natural world that over the long course of human history have advanced health and well-being;
2 foster positive and sustained engagement with natural features and processes;
3 nurture an emotional attachment to particular landscapes and places;
4 promote positive interactions of people with one another and with the natural environment;
5 emphasize interconnected and mutually reinforcing forms of contact with nature, with each application contributing to the overall functioning of a created and designed human ecosystem.

The biophilic design of healthcare facilities should foster an experience of nature that contributes to patient comfort, satisfaction and treatment, the enhanced performance and productivity of healthcare personnel, and promotes the operational effectiveness and efficiency of the institution. The application of biophilic design to healthcare facilities will, nonetheless, inevitably vary depending on particular situational circumstances, opportunities, costs, and constraints.

A range of biophilic design tools or strategies have been developed, and can be roughly divided into three types – the direct experience of nature, indirect contact with natural forms and processes, and characteristics of space and place. The direct experience of nature involves actual contact in the built environment with natural features and forces such as sunlight, air, plants, animals, water, landscapes, and more. *Indirect contact with nature* refers to the representation or image of nature, the transformation of natural materials, and particular patterns and processes of the natural world humans developed an affinity for over evolutionary time. Examples include artwork and pictures of nature, natural material furnishings such as wood and stone, ornamentation inspired by shapes and forms found in the natural world, and such natural processes as organized complexity, fractal geometry, and more. Finally, the characteristics of space and place refers to spatial features of the natural environment of particular relevance to humans such as, for example, an affinity for prospect and refuge, the former because over evolutionary time it assisted people in locating food and water and identifying sources of danger and, the latter, because it contributed to safety and security.

Related to these three categories of biophilic design are a number of specific design strategies that have been identified, although as noted, the choice of which to apply inevitably varies depending on circumstances and constraints. Also as emphasized, the choice of particular design applications should be mutually reinforcing, seeking to create an integrated whole or human ecosystem. With these cautions in mind, the following specific biophilic design applications are as follows:

Direct experience of nature

1 Visual experience of nature. Sight is the dominant sensory means by which humans experience the natural world. This occurs through views to the outside or visual contact with water, plants, animals, landscapes, and other natural features. Aesthetically appealing nature can enhance people's interest, curiosity, imagination, and creativity. Lacking visual contact with nature such as windowless spaces or aesthetically displeasing nature, people are often bored, frustrated, and emotionally and cognitively impaired.

2 Multisensory experience of nature. Other sensory experiences of nature include sound, touch, taste, smell, and motion. Multisensory contact with nature can enhance motivation and comfort, relieve stress, and promote better performance. Touching plants, hearing water or animal sounds, and

smelling flowers can be both restful and stimulating. Conversely, unnatural sensory stimulation such as loud mechanical sounds are often disturbing and debilitating.

3 Light. The experience of natural light, or artificial light that mimics the dynamic and spectral qualities of natural light, foster physical and mental well-being. Access to natural light is especially satisfying, while artificial lighting that simulates the warm, cool, and dynamic properties of natural light is most beneficial. Diffuse and variable light can also evoke the dynamic and sculptural qualities of natural light.

4 Air. Natural atmospheric conditions such as outside ventilation, airflow, and thermal comfort enhance health and well-being. Natural and clean air, comfortable humidity and temperature levels, variable airflow can contribute to enjoyment and satisfaction. This can be achieved through engineering or access to outside conditions such as operable windows.

5 Vegetation. Vegetation and flowering plants often contribute to comfort, reduce stress, and improve performance. Single or isolated plants typically exert little effect. Vegetation in the built environment should be abundant and ecologically connected. Native rather than exotic plants are preferable, and invasive species should be avoided.

6 Animals. The experience of animal life such as fish in an aquarium, birds in an aviary or at feeders, butterflies in a garden, can be emotionally and intellectually pleasing and restorative. This can be achieved through enclosures, tanks, cameras, video, and creative landscape design.

7 Water. Water is basic to life and its positive experience in the built environment can relieve stress, enhance comfort, and promote cognitive functioning. The human affinity for water is multi sensory involving sight, sound, touch, taste, and movement. The experience of water can be achieved through fountains, constructed wetlands, and other strategies.

8 Landscapes. Certain landscapes have been important in human evolution such as savannah settings that include spreading vegetation, an open understory, and the presence of water. Even non-spectacular natural scenery, such as a grove of trees or grass, can be restorative.

9 Natural systems. Self-sustaining natural systems that support an array of environmental features and processes are often satisfying. This can occur through access to outdoor areas, or with sufficient care can be creatively designed such as a native ecosystem or green roof.

Indirect experience of nature

1 Representational images of nature. The image and representation of nature can be emotionally and intellectually satisfying. This can be achieved through photographs, paintings, sculptures, and other images and symbols of plants, animals, water, geological features, and landscapes.

2   Natural materials. Materials that involve the transformation of nature occur in furnishings, flooring, fabrics, and more. Prominent natural materials include wood, stone, wool, cotton, and leather. These materials are visually and tactilely satisfying, revealing the dynamic properties of organic growth in response to environmental forces over time.

3   Natural Colours. Colour is an attribute of people's adaptive reaction to the natural world that over evolutionary time has assisted in locating food and water, aiding movement, and way finding. Earth tones and hues can be especially satisfying.

4   Organic shapes and forms. Some of the most appealing shapes and forms are inspired by elements and features of the natural world. A fabric, decoration, or sometimes even the shape of an entire building can suggest the wings of a bird, the contours of a plant, the geometry of a shell.

5   Movement and mobility. An essential condition of human survival has been the ability to navigate diverse settings. The presence of clear pathways and points of entry and egress are especially important, fostering comfort and security, while their absence often results in confusion and claustrophobia.

6   Growth and time. Nature is dynamic and continuously changing. Living and organic forms reflect patterns of growth and efflorescence. People enjoy environments that possess dynamic qualities that reflect adaptation to circumstances, and mimic the organic qualities of growth and change.

Characteristics of space and place

1   Prospect and refuge. Prospect provides visual access to surrounding environments, often achieved through long vistas. Within buildings this can occur by spatial connections among spaces and views to the outside. Refuge is the experience of secure and protected spaces. Especially satisfying places often possess a mix of prospect and refuge.

2   Organized complexity. People covet complexity in natural and human settings because it signals an environment rich in resources and opportunities. Yet, environments too complex can be confusing. What people seek are complex environments that are orderly and organized.

3   Integrated and coherent space. People enjoy settings with clear and discernible boundaries, and where the relationships between spaces possess overall coherence. These spaces foster a sense of familiarity and security.

4   Simulation of natural space. Built environments that possess qualities of exterior settings are especially satisfying. This can be achieved through expansiveness, as well as the application of natural rather than artificial geometries such as curves, sinuous patterns, and avoiding monolithic shapes and forms.

5   Cultural and ecological connection to place. Humans are territorial because over evolutionary time it contributed to the control of resources,

enhanced mobility and security. An attachment to place reflects a territorial propensity and can be achieved through cultural and ecological connection to local settings. Relevant designs include the use of indigenous materials, vernacular forms, and local plants and animals. A sense of place often encourages ecological and cultural conservation.

Redesigning healthcare facilities

This chapter will conclude with some briefly described examples of biophilia and biophilic design in the healthcare field. This presentation should be viewed with caution for two reasons. First, the author's knowledge of the healthcare field is limited, and this will result in the omission of many relevant examples. Second, all those cited offer only partial illustrations of the impact of biophilia and biophilic design as none provide a comprehensive instance of the application of biophilic design in the healthcare field.

Roger Ulrich Studies

Roger Ulrich, a professor of architecture at the Center for Healthcare Building Research at Chalmers University of Technology in Sweden, has been in the forefront of assessing the health and healing impacts of nature in healthcare settings. Related to this examination, Ulrich contributed insightful chapters to our original volumes on Biophilia (1993) and Biophilic Design (2008), where he cited several relevant examples briefly described here.

The first is a frequently referenced study of patients recovering from gall bladder surgery variably exposed to views of nature. Patients were demographically matched and randomly assigned to two types of rooms – those with a window view of trees and vegetation, the others of a brick wall. The nature view patients had significantly better physical, mental and behavioural health outcomes. The researchers reported (1993: 107): 'Patients with the nature window view had shorter post-surgical hospital stays, ...fewer minor post-surgical complications, [and] far fewer negative comments in nurses notes... The wall view patients required far more potent pain killers.' While this important research provides a partial confirmation of the theory of biophilia, it does little in the way of advancing the application of biophilic design beyond underscoring the importance of views of nature.

A second Ulrich study focused on the impact of a biophilic design retrofit of a windowless hospital emergency room. The original emergency room was a largely featureless space lacking windows, having blank walls, filled with artificial furnishings, and devoid of nature. High levels of stress and aggressive behaviour occurred in this room among visitors and between visitors and staff, prompting calls for its redesign. The emergency room retrofit resulted in an attractive and colourful mural of plants and animals in a savannah-like setting, natural material furnishings and carpeting, organically designed fabrics, and potted plants. It remained a windowless room and the experience of nature was largely indirect and representational. Nonetheless, post-occupancy research found a significant decline in stress levels and aggressive behaviour. This study illustrates the importance of even indirect contact with nature, natural materials, and organic shapes and forms in helping to relieve stress and create a more healthful setting.

A third Ulrich study examined the impact of a new psychiatric facility in Gothenburg, Sweden. The building it replaced was monolithic, barren and sensory deprived. By contrast, the new facility contained extensive gardens, plant-filled courtyards and interior spaces, widespread natural light, prospect and refuge spaces, widespread occurrence of organic shapes and forms, and natural materials. Post-occupancy research found a significant decline in hostility and aggression, the use of physical restraints dropping by more than 40 per cent and a 20 per cent decline in compulsory injections used to control aggressive behaviour (Kellert and Finnegan 2011). The calming and emotionally restorative impact of exposure to nature was again demonstrated, although the lack of a systematic approach to the application of biophilic design limits the lessons to be learned from this occurrence.

Yale-New Haven Smilow Cancer Center (New Haven, Connecticut) and Doernbecher Children's Hospital (Portland, Oregon)

Two healthcare facilities that have incorporated nature into their interior spaces are the Yale-New Haven Hospital Smilow Cancer Center in New Haven, Connecticut, and Doernbecher Children's Hospital in Portland, Oregon, both in the United States. At the Smilow Cancer Center, the interior designer, Rosalyn Cama, incorporated several nature-related features including flowing water, extensive planting, a healing garden, tropical aquaria, and widely distributed paintings and photographs of plants, animals and landscapes. At Doernbecher Children's Hospital, whimsical and childlike depictions of birds and other animals, colourful murals, and vegetation occurred throughout the facility. At both hospitals, anecdotal evidence indicated contact with nature exerted significant stress-relieving effects on patients and visitors alike, and contributed to staff satisfaction and morale. Still, the lack of an overall biophilic design strategy in both instances, and little focus on the external environment, limits the lessons to be learned from these applications.

Khoo Teck Puat Hospital, Singapore

An ambitious attempt at integrating nature into a hospital setting is Khoo Teck Puat Hospital in Singapore. The hospital was conceived from the outset as a 'hospital in a garden, a garden in a hospital,' where 70 per cent of the 12 hectare site was designed to include gardens, verdant open spaces, and water features (Chan 2013). The hospital complex includes an astonishing variety of plants and animals, diverse terrestrial and aquatic habitats, and thousands of identified species of birds, fish, butterflies, flowering plants and other wild animals and vegetation, as well as extensive cultivated flowers and edible and medicinal plants. The hospital has also opened its natural areas to the surrounding community, establishing a highly successful urban farm and creating a strong sense of place.

Khoo Teck Puat Hospital is an impressive accomplishment from the perspective of bringing nature into a hospital setting. Yet, the evidence of its healing, therapeutic, and operational impacts is limited and largely anecdotal. Moreover, from a design perspective, the overall biophilic approach seems somewhat fragmented. No comprehensive biophilic design strategy appeared to guide this effort or its intended health outcomes. The prevailing assumption appeared to be that any contact with nature is beneficial, with the result being a confusing array of design interventions with uncertain impacts. Additionally, contact with nature seemed to be largely confined to the direct experience of the outside environment with little approach to the biophilic design of interior spaces.

Conclusions

Theory and evidence have been cited in support of the theory of biophilia that humans possess inherent affinities for nature and natural processes that continue to exert significant physical and mental health and well-being effects. This apparent demonstration has enormous implications for the practice of medicine and the design of healthcare facilities and associated landscapes.

This chapter identified a framework for the biophilic design of healthcare facilities. This design framework should not be applied, however, in a fragmented and checklist fashion, but rather by seeking to create an integrated and mutually reinforcing whole. Like any organism, humans function best in ecosystems that consist of linked and complementary elements where the emergent whole is greater than the sum of its parts. Not all contact with nature is necessarily biophilic. An isolated planter, a sterile water feature, or a single picture typically exert few if any health impacts. The biophilic design of healthcare facilities should be engaging, ongoing, coherent, and integrated.

A brief review of examples of biophilia and biophilic design in existing healthcare settings provided some important lessons and precedents. None rose to the level, however, of a model of what can be achieved. The effective biophilic design of healthcare facilities should be guided by the principles and design strategies outlined here, and include an empirical assessment of the health and operational impacts of these interventions. A potentially revolutionary change in the design of healthcare facilities may be at hand, one that recognizes how much the human body, mind, and spirit remains deeply contingent on the quality of its connections to the world beyond ourselves of which we remain a part.

Chapter 3

Green exercise for health

A dose of nature

Jo Barton, Carly Wood, Jules Pretty and Mike Rogerson

Introduction

A strong body of evidence now shows that exposure to nature has positive health and well-being benefits. Nature promotes stress recovery, protects from future stresses and improves concentration and ability to think clearly. It is also well established that regular physical activity has both physical and psychological health benefits. Therefore, knowing that both physical activity and nature independently enhance health, the term *Green Exercise* was coined to signify the synergistic health benefits derived from being active in green or natural places (Pretty et al., 2005).

Here we describe theories linking nature and health which underpin the green exercise concept. We then summarise some of the key green exercise research findings to date and discuss the notion of an 'optimal dose' of green exercise for maximum health gain. We identify what further research is required to inform the optimum dose and associated prescriptive guidelines to influence future policy decisions. This chapter mainly focuses on psychological outcomes.

Theories linking nature, green exercise and health

For many thousands of years humans have had regular engagement with nature; from their roles as hunter-gatherers and farmers to, in more recent times, actively seeking natural spaces to reduce the stress of modern life (Fawcett and Gullone, 2001). Whilst research seems to support the biophilia hypothesis discussed in Chapter 2 (Kellert and Wilson, 1993; Kahn, 1997; White and Heerwagen, 1998; Fawcett and Gullone, 2001; Joye, 2007; Grinde and Patil, 2009; Windhager et al., 2011), it is unclear exactly how it might work, which genetic mechanisms are involved and how they are affected by behaviours and external environments.

The ecological dynamics approach offers explanation for how green exercise improves psychological well-being. Compared to synthetic environments, nature environments provide more challenging, complex, varied and intense affordances (invitations or possibilities) (Brymer and Davids, 2012; 2014), whereby individuals can experience a broad range of emotions and other psychological feelings such as mindfulness, peace and calm (Brymer and Davids, 2014).

The Psycho-Evolutionary Stress Reduction theory hypothesises that exposure to nature promotes stress recovery (Ulrich, 1981; Herzog and Strevey, 2008; Ewert et al., 2011). Natural environments provide positive distractions from daily stresses and invoke feelings of interest, pleasantness and calm, thereby reducing stress symptoms and promoting positive affect (Ulrich, 1981, 1984; Herzog and Strevey, 2008; Ewert et al., 2011). This stress reduction restores an individual's physical and mental well-being through affective or emotional changes. Studies supporting this theory report reductions in stress measures such as blood pressure, heart rate and stress hormones following exposure to nature (Ulrich 1991, 1993; Hartig et al., 1996, 2003; Laumann et al., 2003; Herzog and Strevey, 2008; Ward Thompson et al., 2012). The Attention Restoration Theory (Kaplan and Kaplan, 1989; Kaplan, 1995) defines two types of attention: directed attention and involuntary attention. Directed attention requires mental effort and concentration and if overused leads to directed attention fatigue (Kaplan, 1995; Taylor et al., 2002; Berman et al., 2008; Herzog and Strevey, 2008; Taylor and Kuo, 2009; Ewert et al., 2011; Rogerson and Barton, 2015). We regularly engage in this type of attention in everyday lives, often resulting in mental fatigue. However, natural environments promote the use of involuntary attention, providing an opportunity for recovery from mental fatigue (Berman et al., 2008; Taylor and Kuo, 2009; Rogerson and Barton, 2015). For example, Ottoson and Grahn (2005) reported that resting for one hour in an outdoor garden resulted in greater improvements in directed attention than equivalent rest indoors; whilst nature views or the presence of plants within the workplace have been demonstrated to reduce mental fatigue (Kaplan, 1993; Berto, 2005; Raanaas et al., 2011).

Physical activity has also been linked with attention restoration via the transient hypofrontality hypothesis (Dietrich and Sparling, 2004; Dietrich, 2006; Rogerson and Barton, 2015). This suggests that directed attention is associated with prefrontal cortex activation and that physical activity results in prefrontal cortex restoration; as activation of the prefrontal cortex lessens in order to facilitate greater activation of the brain structures concerned with movement (Daffner et al., 2000; Miller and Cohen, 2001; Dietrich and Sparling, 2004; Dietrich, 2006; Rogerson and Barton, 2015). Whilst this decreased prefrontal cortex activity may be detrimental to cognition during physical activity (Dietrich and Sparling, 2004; Labelle et al., 2013) the opportunity for restoration is likely to result in improved executive function and cognitive performance following physical activity (Yangisawa et al., 2010; Byun et al., 2014). Considering the individual benefits of both physical activity and contact with nature for cognition, green exercise provides greater opportunities for restoration due to interaction of the two disparate influences (Rogerson and Barton, 2015). This interaction might account for the additive psychological health benefits of green exercise.

Green exercise research approaches

Green exercise research has predominantly adopted three methodological approaches: (i) comparing outcomes of built versus nature-based outdoor exercise (Hartig et al., 2003; Berman et al., 2008; Park et al., 2010; Lee et al., 2011; Brown et al., 2014); (ii) comparing outcomes of indoor exercise to those of outdoor exercise (Teas et al., 2007; Focht, 2009; Ryan et al., 2010; Thompson Coon et al., 2011); (iii) employing ergometers in laboratory settings to control the exercise component and examine the importance of the visual exercise environment (Pretty et al., 2005; Akers et al., 2012; Wood et al., 2013a; Rogerson and Barton, 2015).

Urban/built versus nature-based outdoor exercise

The main strength of this research is that it represents an ecologically valid comparison, in that individuals may often exercise in one of these two environments. Therefore, such research findings can be understood and applied to real-world settings. The workplace offers a typical contextual example. Brown et al. (2014) asked office workers to undertake two lunchtime walks per week for eight weeks using one of two routes; while some of the office workers always walked a nature route (centered around trees, maintained grass, and public footpaths), others walked a built route (pavements around housing estates and industrial areas). Self-reported mental health improved for those who completed the eight weeks of nature walking, but significant improvements did not occur in the built environment. Berman et al. (2008) found that although walking in a downtown environment and a botanical garden both facilitated improvements in directed attention (a measure that might be described as a psychological resource for, or temporal ability of concentration), the improvement after botanical garden walking was statistically significant; however, the improvement via downtown walking was not. Additionally, walking in a botanical garden elicited greater mood improvements compared to walking in the downtown environment. These results suggest mood and cognitive attention benefit from nature-based exercise environments. Other built versus nature-based walking studies report similar results (Hartig et al., 2003).

A review by Bowler et al. (2010) reported that exercise in natural, compared to man-made, environments was associated with lower negative emotions such as anger and sadness and greater levels of attention. Mitchell (2013) found that people who regularly used the natural environment for physical activity (defined as at least once per week) had about half the risk of poor mental health compared to those who did not do so. Additionally, each extra weekly use of the natural environment for physical activity was identified to reduce the risk of poor mental health by a further 6 per cent. Walking in natural environments compared to environments lacking nature was found to be associated with less perceived stress and negative effect and more positive well-being (Roe and Aspinall, 2011; Marselle et al., 2013). Evidence also suggests that green exercise results in greater improvements in self-esteem and mood, via reductions in tension, depression, anger and confusion and increases in vigour (Barton et al., 2009; Rogerson et al., 2015) and reduced levels of frustration and arousal and higher levels of meditation (Aspinall et al., 2013).

Individuals' choices of built or nature exercise environments may also be important to physiological health outcomes (Li et al., 2011; Lee et al., 2012; Brown et al., 2014). However, these are not discussed here as this topic receives greater attention in Chapters 8 (Li) and 13 (Gladwell and Brown). Despite the merits of this methodological approach, a main limitation is that it often lacks rigorous control of the exercise component, which is important, as exercise characteristics such as duration and intensity themselves influence a number of outcomes (Ekkekakis and Petruzzello, 1999; Ekkekakis et al., 2011).

Indoor versus outdoor exercise

In comparisons of indoor and outdoor activities, it is often difficult to ensure comparability of the exercise component; therefore, it is challenging to infer respective contributions to reported outcomes, of environmental differences and exercise differences. In a review of studies comparing indoor and outdoor physical activity, Thompson Coon et al. (2011) found that compared with walking indoors, outdoor walking was associated with more positive mood, increased self-esteem, vitality, energy and pleasure; alongside reductions in frustration, worry, confusion, depression and tiredness. Running outside was also associated with less anxiety, depression, anger and hostility than running indoors (Thompson Coon et al., 2011). Consistent with this, Focht (2009) found that female participants experienced greater pleasant affective states after an outdoor walk compared to an equivalent indoor walk. They also enjoyed the outdoor walks more and reported a greater intention to continue this behaviour in the future. Such findings are of note for policy-makers in public health, as this suggests a role for green exercise in increasing physical activity participation levels, in utilizing links between affective responses to exercise, intentions, and future exercise behaviours (Williams et al., 2008; Kwan and Bryan, 2010a; 2010b; Ekkekakis et al., 2011).

Ryan et al. (2010) controlled the speed of walking exercise and prohibited verbal social interaction during a comparison of indoor (whereby participants were led through a series of underground hallways and tunnels that were devoid of living things, although there were many objects, posters, physical changes, and colours present) versus outdoor walks (participants led along a largely tree-lined footpath along a river). Greater improvements in feelings of vitality were reported in the outdoors condition, suggesting that exercise environments are important beyond their potential influences on physical exercise and on social interactions. However, the environment may influence social experiences of exercise sessions. Teas et al. (2007) noted that in addition to promoting significantly greater improvements in mood compared to indoor exercise (in a sample of post-menopausal women), outdoor exercise also facilitated participants' engagement in verbal interaction during group exercise. Importantly, this suggested that there are additional social benefits to be gained from green exercise participation in groups.

Urban/Built versus nature views in the laboratory

The strength of this approach is that the exercise component can be rigorously controlled. The limitation is that it does not provide the full-sensory experience of green exercise participation; therefore, it requires further investigation so as to conclude whether laboratory-based findings are fully applicable to the real world.

Pretty et al. (2005) analysed the effect of exercising on a treadmill whilst viewing either rural pleasant, urban pleasant, rural unpleasant or urban unpleasant scenes on self-esteem, mood and blood pressure. There was also an exercise-only condition whereby participants exercised whilst viewing a blank screen. Whilst exercise alone resulted in improvements in self-esteem and mood, viewing urban and rural pleasant scenes during exercising produced greater effects. The unpleasant scenes had a depressive effect on both self-esteem and mood. The response patterns for physiological health outcomes displayed a similar pattern. Blood pressure improved immediately following participation in the exercise-only condition, but significant improvements were only reported after viewing rural pleasant scenes. Exercise whilst viewing the urban unpleasant scenes increased blood pressure relative to the control condition and, therefore, seemed to undo the beneficial effects of exercise for blood pressure (Pretty et al., 2005).

Akers et al. (2012) similarly focused on the role of the visual exercise environment on the outcome of mood, during cycling exercise. After viewing colour-filtered scenes of a first-person movement through a woodland road environment (in a counter-balanced order) during moderate intensity cycling, participants reported greatest improvements in mood following the unedited 'green' video, compared to achromatic- (grey) filtered and red-filtered video. Participants' perceived exertion was also lowest in the unedited video condition, suggesting that environmental colour may contribute to the reported psychological benefits of green exercise. Other research using this methodology reported that during treadmill exercise, compared with viewing either a blank screen, video footage of a built environment or viewing video footage of a nature environment facilitated restoration of depleted directed attention (Rogerson and Barton, 2015). This finding complements the findings of Berman et al. (2008) and Hartig et al. (2003), demonstrating the way in which findings from different methodologies together contribute to a greater understanding of this topic. Again focusing on treadmill exercise, Wood et al. (2013a) found that manipulation of environmental scenes viewed during exercise did not significantly influence self-esteem and mood outcomes in a sample of adolescents, suggesting that age may be an important variable to consider in applications of green exercise.

Is there an 'optimum dose' of green exercise?

Although many physiological outcomes of green exercise have been reported, we will focus here more on psychological outcomes. In order to maximise potential benefits from green exercise participation, it is necessary to know the optimal 'dose' of this experience. This applies equally for either particular outcome measures alone, or for combined mental and physiological health outcomes overall. Dose–response modelling is an analytical technique often used for informing guidelines for health interventions (Shanahan et al., 2015). The effects of different doses of an activity (or substance) on causally linked health responses are modelled; that is, shown by a curve on a graph (Altshuler, 1981; Shanahan et al., 2015). To date, very little research has directly sought to identify optimal characteristics for maximising desired outcomes of green exercise participation (Barton and Pretty, 2010; Rogerson et al., 2015).

A meta-analysis (n=1252) (Barton and Pretty, 2010) revealed distinct dose–response curves for the optimal duration, intensity and types of green exercise activities. For each outcome measure of interest (e.g. mood), a dose–response curve was calculated for each 'dose' variable upon which the measure was assessed (e.g. duration). Figure 3.1 shows curves for the outcome measures of self-esteem and overall mood for the 'dose' variable of duration. This indicates that the greatest benefits to mood and self-esteem occur within the first five minutes of exposure. However, these results may also represent differences in activity type, as this research focuses on a range of different activities (e.g. cycling, walking, gardening, fishing, etc.). Figure 3.2 suggests that for overall mood and self-esteem, 'light' intensity exercise may be most beneficial.

Green exercise participation comprises interactions between numerous environmental, exercise and individual-related variables (Figure 3.3) (Brymer et al., 2014; Rogerson et al., 2015). Therefore, knowledge of optimal doses of exercise per se and of nature exposure might also be considered together with green exercise research findings when attempting to identify an optimal dose of green exercise for health benefits. The three dose–response components for both nature and exercise would include: (i) intensity of exposure [i.e. quality (species richness, biodiversity, habitats, vegetation structure, etc.) and quantity (extent and type of vegetation) of nature]. The quantity and quality of available

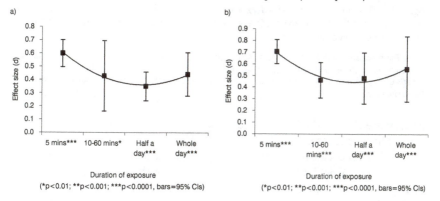

Figure 3.1 a: Dose response data for the effect of exposure duration on self-esteem. b: Dose response data for the effect of exposure duration on Total Mood Disturbance (TMD) (Barton and Pretty, 2010)

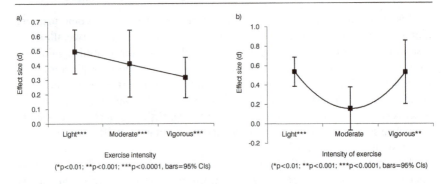

Figure 3.2 a: Dose response data for the effect of exercise intensity on self-esteem. b: Dose response data for the effect of exercise intensity on Total Mood Disturbance (TMD) (Barton and Pretty, 2010)

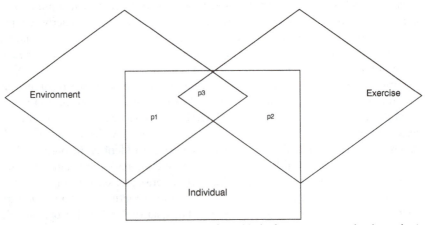

Figure 3.3 The four components (categories of variables) of green exercise: the three physical components (individual; exercise; environment), and the processes component (pp.1-3) (Source: Rogerson et al., 2015)

Note: The processes component comprises psychological and physiological processes within the individual, in relation to either the environment (p1), the exercise (p2), or both (p3; for example, when running in nature, the stimulus of visual optic flow, as perceived by the individual, is a product of exercise-related motion through the environment)

green space close to the home is correlated with longevity and a decreased risk of mental ill-health (Maas et al., 2006, 2009; Ward Thompson et al., 2012; White et al., 2013). Individual preferences and perceptions may also influence the dose response. This would also relate to the intensity of the exercise; (ii) frequency of exposure [how often you exercise or experience nature in a defined time frame. This may also be influenced by the pattern of exposure (e.g. intermittent, random, cumulative, etc.) and the outcomes measured (e.g. psychological or physiological health – frequent short bouts of nature exposure could cumulatively negate mental fatigue but have minimal impact on physiological health, whereas participating in repeated bouts of exercise over a longer time period might enhance cardiovascular health)]; (iii) duration of exposure [length of time of exercise bout and/or nature exposure].

Dose–response relationships for exercise have also been examined. For example, regarding the outcome measure of 'affect', greater pleasure tends to be experienced by individuals when exercise intensity is below lactate threshold, with supra-threshold intensities eliciting negative affect (Ekkekakis et al., 2011). Additionally, self-selected exercise intensity elicits greater positive affect than when intensity is imposed (Ekkekakis et al., 2011).

The notion of an optimal dose of exposure to nature has also received consideration. Shanahan et al. (2015) reviewed existing literature to analyse the potential shapes of dose–response curves for nature dose (duration of exposure) and a health outcome. They identified four potential shapes: (i) rapid increase after low dosage (e.g. cognitive function improved within 10 minutes of viewing natural images, Berto, (2005)), followed by a plateau; (ii) decline in health parameter (as dosage continues to increase); (iii) a more gradual increase (as dosage increases), followed by a plateau; and (iv) decline in health parameter. Attention restoration theory predicts that different types of nature may offer different scope for psychological restoration, as it is the presence of particular characteristics of nature environments which are important to their influence (for example, fascination; extent) (Kaplan, 1995). Concurrently, different types of nature provide different opportunities, or affordances, for individuals to gain health benefits (Brymer et al., 2014).

The presence of water within environments has been suggested to enhance affective outcomes of nature exposure (White et al., 2010), and this has also been shown to occur via green exercise participation (Barton and Pretty, 2010), although this influence may be less important at higher exercise intensities (Rogerson et al., 2015). Furthermore regarding exposure to nature per se, the 'dose' variables of: number of habitats in a given environment, duration of exposure to nature and overall environment type, have been considered in relation to the 'response' outcome measures of individuals' reflection scores, reductions in blood pressure, and stress reduction, respectively (Shanahan et al., 2015). These dose–response relationships are shown in Figure 3.4.

In order to understand the overall optimal dose across multiple health measures, responses for multiple outcomes (e.g. mental well-being, cognitive function, blood pressure) might be assessed for a given dose variable, in order to identify an average trend. Following calculation of dose–response curves for given outcome measures in relation to different 'dose' variables, these may either be considered disparately, or analysed to examine possible interactions between curves (e.g. duration by exercise intensity interaction). Although it is beyond the scope of the current chapter to calculate what an optimal dose of green exercise might comprise, this may be achieved increasingly accurately as the body of research evidence grows. To enable calculations of optimal green exercise doses, there is a

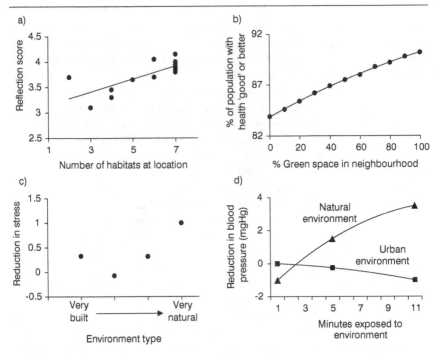

Figure 3.4 Examples of the dose–response relationship between nature and measures of health or well-being from previous studies

(a) psychological well-being ('reflection') in response to exposure to different numbers of habitat types in Sheffield, United Kingdom (Fuller et al. 2007); (b) the change in mean arterial diastolic blood pressure over time during exposure to urban and natural settings in California (adapted from Hartig et al. 2003 to show only the first section of the experiment where participants were not exercising); (c) the change in stress levels in response to different landscape types (adapted from Beil and Hanes 2013 to show inverse of stress measure originally presented) (Source: Shanahan et al., 2015).

need for researchers to present effect sizes for their data, to ensure comparability of results. Furthermore, separate dose–response curves will be required to identify optimal frequency of green exercise behaviours, as opposed to outcomes of acute bouts of green exercise.

In addition to identifying the optimum dose of green exercise, it is important to know *who* that dose may benefit most and least. Barton and Pretty's (2010) meta-analysis found that the health benefits of green exercise were greatest for those with declared mental health problems. Concurrently, Roe and Aspinall (2011) found that people with mental health problems experienced greater reductions in stress following a rural walk than people with a good level of mental health. These findings suggest that green exercise should also play an important role in improving the health and well-being of people suffering from mental ill-health.

More evidence is required for differences in psychological green exercise benefits between sexes to become clear. Whereas Barton and Pretty's (2010) meta-analysis found both women and men similarly to gain benefits from green exercise participation, a more recent study reported that sex significantly explained 6.8 per cent of variance in pre- to post-green exercise mood improvements (Rogerson et al., 2015). Age could also be a mediating factor as improvements in self-esteem declined with age, whilst the improvements in mood followed a U-curve shape with middle-aged participants experiencing the greatest degree of benefits (Barton and Pretty, 2010). Interestingly, influences of exercise environment on self-esteem and mood demonstrated in adult samples have not been found for children (Reed et al., 2013; Wood et al., 2013a). This suggests that age is a factor that should be considered for green exercise interventions.

In addition to individual characteristics, other mediating factors might include specific individual–environmental and exercise-related variables, such as personal preferences, knowledge and memory, previous experiences and perceptions of nature (degree of perceived restorativeness of landscape), enjoyment and nature relatedness (Hartig et al., 2014; Shanahan et al., 2015). Perceived neighbourhood greenness is strongly associated with better mental and physical health; those living in highly green areas are between 1.37 and 1.6 times more likely to have better mental health (Sugiyama et al., 2008). Rogerson et al. (2015) reported that participants who were more connected to nature and who reported greater enjoyment of their green exercise activity experienced the greatest number of health benefits. Culture and socio-economic status may also influence nature provision (i.e. quantity and quality of nature) and the level of engagement with nature (i.e. duration and frequency of nature dose due to different cultural value systems and attachments to landscapes) (Keniger et al., 2013; Shanahan et al., 2015). Increased access to green space is associated with improved general health, regardless of socio-economic status; whilst income-related inequality in health is moderated by exposure to green space (Allen and Balfour, 2014). Ethnicity can also influence attitudes, green-space use and motivation to engage in outdoor recreation (Ozguner, 2011).

Despite this discussion of who may benefit from optimal doses of green exercise, large proportions of the psychological benefits of green exercise appear to be universally obtainable and independent of demographic, performance level, climatic and other environmental characteristics (Rogerson et al., 2015). This indicates that green exercise is a valuable method for improving the health and well-being of a wide variety of different groups of people.

Conclusions

Engaging in green exercise provides a number of benefits for health and well-being including reductions in anxiety and stress; improved mood, self-esteem, attention, concentration and physical health. Natural environments promote physical activity and social contact which in turn also improve health and well-being. A lot of the existing evidence is correlational (Keniger et al., 2013), so in order to develop and promote effective public health interventions an 'optimal dose' of green exercise needs to be identified. This requires an understanding of the types and amounts of nature and exercise needed to maximise health gains. Developing appropriate dose–response curves would inform prescriptive guidelines and minimum dose recommendations similar to existing public health recommendations for physical activity (30 minutes of moderate activity per day, Powell et al., 2011) and fruit and vegetable consumption (five a day).

Although these recommendations are simplistic in their nature they are straightforward to communicate, they provide guidance for self-regulating behaviours that enhance health outcomes and have substantial impact at a population level (Whitelaw, 2012; Hartig et al., 2014). However, dose–response modelling is challenging because it is subjected to many influential factors, such as individual characteristics, personal preferences and experiences, culture and socio-economic status. The dose–response relationship may also differ when considering population or individual level studies. Population response curves could inform urban green space and cost-effective spatial planning to maximise health outcomes. Using an epidemiological approach to develop dose–response curves enables confounding factors to be statistically controlled for but does not explain causality. Experimental studies at an individual level can help to demonstrate causality, but they need to be rigorous in their design and can often lack statistical power.

To date, dose–response modelling has shown the greatest benefits for self-esteem and mood occur after the first five minutes of green exercise, which should be of a light intensity. This represents an important public health message as it is easier to engage sedentary individuals in light intensity exercise of a short duration. Although this will not have an immediate impact on their physical health, engaging individuals in green exercise is often the biggest challenge. The physiological health benefits will accrue as participation continues. Furthermore, green exercise is of most benefit for people with mental ill-health; suggesting that there may be potential for the therapeutic application of green exercise. If future experimental work continues to report effect sizes, then a meta-analysis can be conducted to build on the existing dose–response data. Public health policies can then consider the use of nature and green exercise for improving and preventing ill-health and provide regular opportunities for people to access natural spaces.

Chapter 4

How to get more out of the green exercise experience

Insights from attention restoration theory

Jason Duvall and William C. Sullivan

Introduction

A nagging injury and the approach of winter prompted Emily to join a local gym. At first, it seemed like a great idea. A few of her friends were members, there was lots of fancy exercise equipment, and venturing out into the cold was never something she really looked forward to. Exercise was generally something that Emily enjoyed, but after a few months at the gym working out began to feel more and more like a monotonous chore. While the time she logged on the 'dreadmill' kept her in shape, she didn't feel as mentally refreshed and clearheaded as when she was running outside. In fact, she found herself constantly craving for breaks in the weather so she could escape the gym and get out into nature. This got Emily wondering whether there was something special about exercising in nature. Could outdoor exercise really make her feel better? If so, were there certain types of outdoor settings that might be especially beneficial? She did seem to have lots of good ideas during her runs through the nature preserve. Maybe she should make more of an effort to get outside even when there was a little chill in the air?

At first glance, you might think that Emily's hunches about exercising in green spaces are just wishful thinking. As long as she gets her heart rate up, challenges her body to move with vigour, and does so for at least 30 minutes, why should the setting matter? And why would green settings in particular have any impact on how Emily feels after exercising? But there is mounting evidence that exercising in green spaces may provide significant benefits beyond cardiovascular health. These psychological benefits are wide-ranging and are likely to last for hours after one has showered and returned to other activities.

Consider some recent findings. Compared to their peers who had been randomly assigned to windowless classrooms or classrooms with windows opening to a built space, high school students assigned to classrooms with windows that opened on to a green space scored significantly higher on standard tests of attention (Li and Sullivan, in press). Compared to seeing scenes of an urban setting without vegetation, viewing scenes of a green space or a forest significantly reduces the stress people feel (Brown et al., 2013; Jiang et al., 2014).

We consider here what might promote such findings, examine additional recent results regarding the benefit of exposure to nature on well-being and pose some suggestions for individuals to ponder as they make decisions about where to exercise.

Attention Restoration Theory

There is powerful evidence that contact with green spaces helps restore and replenish a resource that is essential to functioning in our modern world: our ability to pay attention (Kaplan and Kaplan, 1989; Kaplan, 1995). Our ability to pay attention is one of the most important and useful resources humans possess. We use it constantly – indeed, you are using it now as you read this chapter. We use our attention to accomplish nearly everything that is important to us. It is a requirement for planning, problem-solving, negotiating, setting goals, monitoring and regulating behaviour, and engaging in effective social interactions.

Humans have two modes of absorbing and attending to information. Some objects, ideas, settings, and situations are effortlessly engaging and require no work as we take them in. Kaplan and Kaplan (1989) call this mode *involuntary attention*. It takes no effort, for instance, to watch a fire, look at a waterfall, or gaze at the birds in the trees outside your window. Indeed, it is difficult *not* to pay attention to some things: a toddler who is approaching the stairs, a story of someone being cheated, a deer or fox or other wild creature immediately outside your home.

Other stimuli and settings oblige us to focus on the matter at hand, that is, they require us to pay attention – or as the Kaplans say, to *direct attention*. Unfortunately, our capacity to direct attention is finite. As most people will have likely noticed, after a period of focused concentration – writing a proposal, planning a budget, an intense effort to complete a project – our capacity to focus our attention diminishes. After a period of intense use, our capacity to deliberately direct attention declines.

The costs of attentional fatigue (often called mental fatigue) are profound and far-reaching; they include becoming inattentive, withdrawn, irritable, distractible, impulsive, and accident-prone. This is certainly not a welcome state, but one that is strikingly familiar to all of us who lead busy lives. The good news is that some places have the capacity to alleviate mental fatigue and help restore a person's capacity to pay attention. Such places seem to have in common four characteristics.

Restorative settings

Think for a moment of a time when you were mentally fatigued – perhaps after you completed a proposal, organized an event, planned a wedding or perhaps at the end of a normally busy day. Now, imagine a place that would be restorative, a place that would allow you to clear your head and regain your capacity to focus, see things clearly, and feel on top of your game. Attention Restoration Theory (ART) proposes that such a restorative place has four characteristics. We will now consider each.

Being Away. Removing yourself from mentally fatiguing activities is a prerequisite for restoring your capacity to pay attention. Although you could seek out a secluded garden or go to a monastery, deep seclusion is not necessary. Kaplan and Kaplan (1989) have proposed three ways to elicit the sense of being away: eliminate distractions from your surroundings, take a break from your usual work or responsibilities, and cease your pursuit of attentionally demanding tasks or activities. While taking this break, it will help if your surroundings include some gently fascinating characteristics.

Fascination. Fascinating objects or places have at least one thing in common: they require little or no attentional effort. Watching songbirds at a birdfeeder, gazing at a sunset, holding a newborn baby call on involuntary attention and in doing so allow your capacity to direct your attention to rest and recover. While fascinating settings may come in many forms, natural environments seem to be especially rich in fascinating content (Herzog et al., 1997; Kaplan and Kaplan, 1989).

Think for a moment about taking a run along the edge of a river. Your attention may be called to the movement of the water, the sounds of birds, the play of light and shade on the path, the feel of the breeze on your skin. These stimuli are a gentle form of fascination – soft fascination – that holds your attention without demanding it the way television programmes, video games, or a sporting content most often do. When you are engaged with softly fascinating stimuli your attention is held in such a way as to leave some capacity to examine some of the thoughts that have been running around in your head – thoughts, for instance, about the challenges or opportunities you are facing. Softly fascinating settings foster a deeply beneficial restorative experience (Kaplan et al., 1998; Herzog et al., 2011a).

Extent. Restorative settings contain a feeling of extent, or the sense of being in a place with sufficient scope that one can dwell there for a while. The place need not be vast but it should have enough latitude to engage one's mind. A walk in a restored prairie or in the woods can provide a sense of extent. So can working in one's garden. The key to extent is that the setting be either physically, or conceptually large enough and coherent enough to allow your mind to drift into it. This process of allowing your thoughts to drift away from your daily activities into something that is rich and non-threatening seems an important part of a restorative experience that exercise in green settings can often provide.

Compatibility. Compatibility concerns the extent to which a setting supports a person's inclinations, needs, and purpose in the moment. Compatibility involves the fit between what you are trying to accomplish in the moment and the kind of activities supported, encouraged, or demanded by the place you occupy (Herzog et al., 2003, 2011a, 2011b). Take for instance a person who needs a break from planning an event. She could sit in her office and surf the Internet or she could take a walk in the park by her office. The latter choice is likely to be far more compatible with her goal of taking a break than the former.

Kaplan and Kaplan have observed that these four characteristics of restorative places (being away, fascination, extent, and compatibility) are often available in green settings. ART predicts that contact with green landscapes – even in cities –

should assist in recovery from mental fatigue (Kaplan and Kaplan, 1989; Kaplan, 1995). If that is the case, then gaining exposure to natural settings on a regular basis, even natural elements in urban areas, should have a positive impact on attention restoration. Is there evidence in support of such predictions?

Benefits of nature-based restorative settings

An extensive body of empirical evidence has accumulated in support of ART: exposure to green settings consistently boosts a person's capacity to pay attention. The findings come from green settings, such as forests (Park et al., 2010), rural areas (Roe and Aspinall, 2011), community parks (Fuller et al., 2007), schools (Li and Sullivan, in press; Matsuoka, 2010), neighbourhoods (Rappe and Kivela, 2005), and laboratory settings (Berto, 2005; Rogerson and Barton, 2015). Even short exposures to green spaces result in fewer errors and better ability to focus attention (Lee et al., 2015). Studies have demonstrated links between green spaces and higher performance on attentional tasks in public housing residents, AIDS caregivers, cancer patients, college students, prairie restoration volunteers, and employees of large organizations (for an overview, see Sullivan, 2015).

Perhaps most strikingly, children diagnosed with attention-deficit hyperactivity disorder (ADHD) have been found to benefit from exposure to urban parks and other green spaces near their homes. In a series of studies, such access has been consistently linked with a reduction in ADHD symptoms (Taylor et al., 2001; Kuo and Taylor, 2004; Taylor and Kuo, 2009). Children with ADHD concentrated significantly better after a walk in a park than after a downtown walk or a walk in a neighbourhood (Taylor and Kuo, 2009).

Reflection as an additional benefit

The soft fascination that characterizes natural environments hints at another potential benefit of green exercise – namely, the opportunity to reflect and gain perspective on life issues. According to ART, the soft fascination often found in nature does not completely overwhelm our attentional system, unlike say watching a television programme. In other words, when we're immersed in softly fascinating nature content we are not completely swept away – we still have the mental room in our heads to think about other things (Kaplan, 1995).

Others have suggested that natural content may promote neural activity that encourages a more contemplative and less egocentric frame of mind. According to Kaufman (2015) nature interactions may lead to the activation of neural networks that support subconscious processing and cognitive flexibility. Anecdotally, the notion that nature can encourage these types of reflective states makes a good deal of sense. In fact, many of us make an effort to seek out the tranquil beauty of nature when we need to contemplate life or just decompress after a long day. There is also empirical evidence supporting this idea. Researchers have found that people have an easier time resolving minor life problems while spending time in natural settings (Mayer et al., 2008). In addition, when people are asked about the types of settings most supportive of reflection they express a strong preference for natural environments (Herzog et al., 1997).

It is important to note that the reflection referred to here is different than rumination – the tendency to get stuck pondering on one's situation. Rumination is a maladaptive pattern of repeatedly engaging in a thought. It is associated with heightened risk for depression and other mental illnesses. But a recent study found that walking in a natural setting decreases both self-reported rumination and neural activity associated with rumination, whereas a walk in an urban setting had no such effects (Bratman et al., 2015). This suggests that nature-based activity may not only give people an opportunity to hear what's on their mind, think through everyday problems, and evaluate life decisions, but it might also help shut down negative and persistent internal thoughts.

Restoration and the Human-Nature Interaction

The ability to identify features of restorative environments may lead one to believe that gaining psychological benefits is merely a matter of selecting the correct setting for green exercise. There is, of course, an element of truth to this assumption. Some settings clearly do a better job of encouraging us to set aside demanding tasks and contain greater amounts of softly fascinating stimuli than others. Seeking out and being active in these sorts of environments should result in better restorative outcomes. This notion, however, ignores an important and often underappreciated aspect of ART – namely that how one chooses to interact with the setting also matters (Kaplan, 1995; Kaplan, 2001).

The importance of the human-nature interaction might be most easily seen with respect to the issue of compatibility. As previously described, a compatible environment supports one's goals and intentions; it helps us accomplish the tasks and activities we want to carry out. This indicates that restoration is more likely to occur when there is a match between our purposes and the affordances offered by the environment. For instance, if our goal is to take a leisurely walk outside, then an environment that is easy to navigate and has well-maintained walking paths has enormous restorative potential. However, the restorative potential of this same setting may be greatly reduced if storm clouds roll in and it begins to rain. If we continued to pursue our goal of taking a walk under these incompatible conditions many of us would be more likely to experience frustration rather than restoration. In these circumstances altering our plans is often necessary if we hope to gain restorative benefits (e.g., we could decide to sit on the porch, watch the rain, and walk later).

As with compatibility, the ability of the environment to facilitate being away can also be influenced by how one chooses to interact with the setting. Escaping to a remote and tranquil natural setting is likely to do little good if one decides to bring along demanding work or dwell on old problems. Alternatively, it is possible to feel miles away from daily demands without going all that far provided one has the right mindset. The restorative qualities of extent and fascination too are impacted by the nature of our interactions with the environment. Being preoccupied with external and/or internal distractions can cause us to overlook the less obvious richness that can often exist in mundane or highly familiar natural settings and these same distractions can prevent us from seeing fascinating content that is more obscure. In order to appreciate this, one simply needs to think about an instance of being drawn to some discrete feature of the environment only to discover a whole host of other intriguing elements that were previously invisible.

To be clear, this does not mean all settings are inherently equal in restorative potential, but it does suggest that the way one engages (or fails to engage) with the environment can enhance or interfere with restorative outcomes. In terms of green exercise, this insight raises a number of interesting and highly researchable questions about how to get more out of outdoor physical activity. The remainder of this section examines a number of activities that may undermine restorative benefits and then explores a promising strategy for heightening the restorative experience.

Common activities that may interfere with restoration

Getting an exercise routine going and keeping it going can be a big challenge. As a result, people incorporate all sorts of other activities in an effort to make the exercise experience less tedious and more enjoyable. Traditionally this might have involved working out with a partner or listening to music, but now, with advances in digital technologies, this can include making phone calls, texting, tweeting, and sending email while exercising.

Before discussing the drawbacks that might be associated with these sorts of interest-enhancing activities in terms of restoration, it is important to acknowledge that many of these strategies do have benefits. There is ample evidence, for instance, that walking with a partner can help one initiate and maintain a physical activity routine (Dishman et al., 1985; Sherwood and Jeffery, 2000). Listening to music while exercising has also been associated with positive outcomes, such as improved mood and reduced feelings of physical fatigue (Karageorghis and Priest, 2008; Razon et al., 2009). We make this point to emphasize that none of the interesting-enhancing strategies mentioned above are inherently 'bad', in fact, many are extremely valuable for promoting physical activity. That said, there is reason to believe that some of these activities may encourage interactions that tax attentional resources and/or hinder our ability to notice restorative features of the green exercise environment.

Activities such as talking on a mobile phone or texting require us to both track what is going on and to respond in an appropriate way. Accomplishing these tasks draws on the finite and fatigable resource of directed attention and forces us to shift our attentional focus away from the external environment. Studies examining walking behaviour are consistent with this view, suggesting that mobile phone use increases cognitive demands and reduces situational awareness (Hyman et al., 2010; Lamberg and Muratori, 2012; Lim et al., 2015). These same demands are also likely to be present when exercising with a partner since again, attention must be dedicated to monitoring conversation and detecting social cues. While this relationship has not been extensively examined, several studies indicate that in safe, predictable natural settings walking alone actually results in better restorative outcomes (Staats and Hartig, 2004; Johansson et al., 2011). Presumably, listening to music presents similar challenges. The introduction of auditory stimuli competes for attention with external environmental stimuli making one less sensitive to the world around us.

While restorative outcomes likely vary depending on how these interest-enhancing activities are carried out, it seems reasonable to suggest that engaging in these sorts of tasks may make it difficult for us to truly be away from attentional demands and notice the softly fascinating features so prevalent in natural environments. What's more, these activities may limit opportunities for reflection by making it harder for us to hear what's on our mind.

Strategies for enhancing the restorative experience

If activities that divide our attention and prevent us from being fully present can undermine restoration, then perhaps restoration can be enhanced by performing activities that help us focus and tune in to the natural environment. Kaplan (2001) has lent support to this idea by proposing that greater restoration should result from cognitive engagement with the environment. Although research into this area is still in its early stages, findings from several studies have indicated that heightening environment awareness might be associated with more positive restorative outcomes.

Lin et al. (2014) investigated the impact increasing levels of awareness have on restoration within urban streetscapes. In this study participants were randomly assigned to four awareness conditions (i.e., none, minimal, moderate, and heightened). Individuals in the no awareness condition were shown a series of images of a streetscape with no vegetation whatsoever. The minimal awareness group was shown the same images but with three very brief flashes (30 milliseconds) of street trees. Participants in the moderate awareness condition were shown the tree lined streetscape images for the entire time. Finally, those assigned to the heightened awareness group were shown the tree lined streetscape and were given explicit instructions to observe the scenes closely. Changes in directed attention capacity were assessed before and after participants were exposed to the streetscape images using a Digit Span Backward Test (DSBT), which requires participants to repeat an increasingly long string of numbers in reverse order. Results indicated that directed attention improved for all participants exposed to green streetscapes; however participants who were explicitly asked to take notice (those in the heightened awareness condition) experienced significantly greater benefits. These findings suggest that efforts to heighten environmental awareness can enhance the restorative experience.

Research by Duvall (2011, 2013) has explored the influence that environmental awareness has on restorative outcomes in the context of green exercise specifically.

In this work individuals interested in adopting an outdoor walking routine were recruited and randomly assigned to either a standard care or environmental engagement condition. Participants in the standard care group were given a goal of taking at least three 30-minute outdoor walks each week during the two-week treatment period. These individuals then developed a personalized walking schedule and made a written commitment to stick with their plan. Participants in the environmental engagement group were given the same overall walking goal, but rather than develop a walking schedule they were given a list of awareness plans, which they were asked to use on each walk during the treatment period. These awareness plans, inspired by Leff (1984), were designed to help individuals be more engaged and attentive to features of the physical environment (see Table 4.1). Restoration was measured by asking participants to rate their attentional functioning, feelings of frustration, and feelings of contentment at the beginning and end of the two-week treatment period. In addition, participants were asked to rate their level of satisfaction with the walking environment.

Results from this work revealed that while participants in the two conditions walked for similar amounts of time, the environmental engagement group experienced more restorative benefits. More specifically, participants asked to use the awareness plans were much more likely to report significant improvements in attentional functioning and significant declines in frustration. There was also some evidence indicating that the awareness plans had more positive impacts on participants who walked at low or moderate levels, raising the possibility that efforts to promote environmental engagement may allow people to gain more restorative benefits from shorter bouts of green exercise.

In addition, the environmental engagement appeared to be more effective at influencing participants' perceptions of the walking environment. Individuals using the awareness plans reported being significantly more satisfied with the diversity of natural features, tree cover, and the availability and condition of walking paths. While this result does not directly relate to restoration, greater satisfaction with the green exercise environment may make one more likely to choose and stick with outdoor activity – thereby increasing the potential for restorative benefits.

Table 4.1 Samples of awareness plans

Plan Category	Example
Focus on your senses	Focus on sounds. If the area is quiet, listen to the silence. If the area is full of sounds, focus on each one and notice how they differ.
Take on a new job or role	Imagine you are an artist looking for beauty in everyday things.
Make guesses or inferences	How would this area change if everyone had to grow their own food?
Use magic	If you could cast spells that changed the environment what would you change?

More research is clearly needed before any definitive statements can be made about how to enhance restorative outcomes though green exercise. However, these intriguing studies suggest that efforts to orient our awareness toward the natural environment may have important advantages over activities that draw our focus away from the green exercise setting. What's more, it appears that encouraging environmental engagement may not be terribly difficult. By selecting a few awareness plans to experiment with before we walk out the door, we may be able to have a more satisfying and restorative green exercise experience.

Conclusions

Like Emily, many of us seem to be vaguely aware of the fact that there's something extra one gets from exercising in nature. This seems to go well beyond just making the exercise experience itself more enjoyable. As we have seen there is substantial empirical evidence indicating that people receive significant psychological benefits from spending time in nature. Not only do we tend to be in a better mood after being outdoors in green spaces, but we are also less mentally fatigued and better able to focus on our work, resolve problems, and be patient and tolerant of others. In addition, we have seen that ART provides a strong theoretical foundation for making sense of these findings and offers important practical suggestions about the type of outdoor settings and the type of human-nature interactions that might help us get even more out of green exercise.

According to ART, green settings that provide us with opportunities for being away, extent, fascination, and compatibility are likely to be associated with stronger restorative outcomes. Restoration may also be enhanced through interactions that help us tune in to the external environment and notice the everyday natural features that surround us. Given this research, perhaps we should be more willing to leave our devices behind and venture outdoors when getting our dose of exercise.

Chapter 5

The benefits of green exercise for children

Carly Wood, Rachel Bragg and Jules Pretty

Introduction

The health benefits of engaging in physical activity during childhood include enhanced fitness, improved bone health and cognitive function, favourable cardiovascular and metabolic disease risk profiles, motor skill development, healthier blood pressure and heart rate, and a reduction in body fat (Janssen and Leblanc, 2010; Janz et al., 2010; World Health Organisation, 2010; Faigenbaum and Myer, 2012; Duncan et al., 2014; Larson et al., 2015). Regular physical activity during youth is also known to enhance psychological health, improving self-esteem and reducing symptoms of anxiety and depression (Calfas and Taylor, 1994; Ekeland et al., 2005). Despite these benefits, approximately 75 per cent of boys and 80 per cent of girls aged 5–10 years in the UK do not perform the recommended daily 60 minutes of moderate to vigorous physical activity (MVPA) (Health and Social Care Information Centre, 2014). This is higher in adolescents aged 11–15 years with 83 per cent of boys and 89 per cent of girls not meeting daily activity requirements (Health and Social Care Information Centre, 2014). Regular participation in physical activity during early and youth years is particularly important as physical activity often tracks into adulthood where adequate levels of physical activity are protective against many chronic diseases.

Evidence suggests that the natural environment can play a role in promoting physical activity in children and young people; encouraging free play, which is essential to their health, wellbeing and development (Bird, 2007; Bowler et al., 2010). In adults, engaging in physical activity whilst exposed to natural environments also provides additive benefits for psychological health compared with physical activity in a non-natural environment or indoors (Pretty et al., 2005; 2007; Barton and Pretty, 2010; Thompson Coon et al., 2011). This chapter discusses the importance of natural environments for facilitating physical activity and spontaneous play in children and young people. It also compares the health benefits of green exercise in children to those evident in adults and assesses potential reasons for any differences. We address the issue of disconnection from nature and how to reconnect children to the outdoors.

The natural environment and physical activity

The natural environment provides a setting for physical activity (Pretty et al., 2005; Bowler et al., 2010). Time spent outdoors is a positive correlate of physical activity in children and adolescents (Gorden-Larsen et al., 2000; Sallis et al., 2000; Cleland et al., 2008; Lachowycz et al., 2012), whilst adults with easy access to natural settings are three times as likely to be active (Wells et al., 2007; Bowler et al., 2010). Lachowycz et al. (2012) found that time spent in green space contributes over one-third of all outdoor physical activity on weekday evenings, over 40 per cent on Saturdays and 60 per cent on Sundays, indicating both that children are high users of green environments and that green space may be an important contributor to overall physical activity levels. In addition, a review of studies examining the relationship between green space use and physical activity found a positive relationship or evidence of an association in two-thirds of children (Lachowycz and Jones, 2011).

The availability of parks and open spaces is positively associated with physical activity in children and adolescents; and are second behind schools as settings where young people are active (Epstein et al., 2006; Loukaitou-Sideris and Sideris, 2009; Mahdjoubi and Spencer, 2010; Floyd et al., 2011; Larson et al., 2015). It has also been shown that the proportion of total park area in a community is a significant predictor of children's physical activity, with physical activity increasing by 1.4 per cent for every 1 per cent increase in park area (Roemmich et al., 2006; Timperio et al., 2008). Approximately 50 per cent of children and young people engage in MVPA whilst in a park area (Floyd et al., 2008a, b); with each extra hour of park use resulting in an extra 35 minutes of MVPA (Larson et al., 2015). Thus, natural settings and particularly local parks and open spaces, may play a key role in promoting physical activity in children and young people (Timperio et al., 2008).

Research comparing physical activity levels in young people during exposure to different types of environments has supported the notion that the natural environment facilitates physical activity. One such study compared physical activity levels during school playtime on the playground and field: playtime on the field resulted in 40 per cent more MVPA than play on the playground (Wood et al., 2014a). Similar findings were also demonstrated in a study comparing activity levels during urban and rural orienteering. Children were significantly more active during rural orienteering, spending half of their time in the natural environment in physical activity compared with only one-quarter in the built environment (Wood et al., 2014b). We are able to conclude that natural environments promote inclusion in physical activity by: i) reducing the gap in the differences in male and female physical activity levels and encouraging girls to be more active (Wood et al., 2014a, b); ii) engaging the less fit children in physical activity (Barton et al., 2014); and iii) making physical activity seem easier and more enjoyable to children who are less physically active (Reed et al., 2013). This combined benefit of physical activity and exposure to green space is likely to be of particular importance in light of the growing concerns over physical inactivity, poor physical and mental health and childhood obesity.

A number of studies have also assessed the impact of living environment on habitual physical activity. Whilst some studies have indicated that children living in rural settings are more active and fitter than those living in urban settings (Dyment and Bell, 2008; Joens-Matre et al., 2008; Liu et al., 2008; Adamo et al., 2012; Liu et al., 2012), others have suggested that there are no differences between the two (Loucaides et al., 2004; Plotnikoff et al., 2004; Sandercock et al., 2010). In some locations, children from urban areas are more active than their rural counterparts (Goran et al., 1998; Bathrellou et al., 2007; Sheu-Jen et al., 2010; Al-Nuaim et al., 2012). The inconsistency between these findings can be attributed to the fact that the studies have focused on the presence of green space in the living environment and not the actual location where the physical activity is performed (Lachowycz et al., 2012; Wood, 2012a). Children living in urban areas may have access to local green space which they use for physical activity, whilst children from rural areas are often close to green space but cannot always access it (Sheu-Jen et al., 2010). Equally, some urban spaces are perceived as unsafe for children and young people, and thus act as a barrier to participation in physical activity (Molnar et al., 2003; Mahdjoubi and Spencer, 2015).

The importance of play in natural spaces

Play has been defined as the spontaneous activity in which children engage to amuse and occupy themselves (Burdette and Whittaker, 2005). However, spontaneous and unregulated play is becoming less common in affluent countries due to parental fears of strangers, the loss of natural spaces for free play, and contrasting perceptions about what is best for children and young people (Louv, 2005; Bird, 2007). The loss of spontaneous free play in natural spaces is particularly concerning, as play in nature is important for the health, wellbeing and development of children. Natural environments are varied and changeable and thus provide good opportunities for free explorative play which gives greater opportunities for decision-making whilst also enabling children to develop the capacity for creativity and symbolic play, both essential for personal and cognitive development (RSPB, 2010; Department for Education, 2013). Furthermore, play in nature can improve concentration, and for children suffering from attention deficit hyperactivity disorder (ADHD) can enable increased functioning and a reduction in the severity of attention deficit symptoms (Taylor et al., 2001; Kuo and Taylor, 2004; Munoz, 2009).

In addition, play in nature has been shown to promote risk-taking, independence and autonomy, and results in positive attitudes towards the environment (Ward Thompson et al., 2006; Bird, 2007; Lester and Maudsley, 2007). Play in nature also promotes physical, social, emotional and cognitive development; improves motor fitness, motor skills, balance and coordination; and produces healthy growth and a good level of mental health (Fjørtoft, 2004;

Munoz, 2009). Through play in nature, children have greater levels of social interactions which promote an aptitude for learning (Pretty et al., 2009; Bragg et al., 2013). They are also provided with an opportunity to develop problem-solving skills, improve their communication, co-operation, interpersonal and decision-making skills, whilst promoting responsibility and imagination (RSPB, 2010). There is also some evidence to suggest that play in nature can reduce bullying and aggressive behaviour (Malone and Tranter, 2003; Mahdjoubi and Spencer, 2015). Thus, the opportunity to play in natural environments may play a key role in promoting individual health and wellbeing in children and young people, as well as stronger communities.

Comparison of green exercise outcomes in youth and adults

Earlier chapters have shown that green exercise in adults provides additive benefits for self-esteem and mood above those received from exercise alone (Pretty et al., 2005; Barton and Pretty, 2010). Despite the well-documented benefits of engaging in green exercise via activities such as outdoor adventure programmes and forest schools (Paxton and McAvoy, 2000; Pryor et al., 2005; O'Brien and Murray, 2007) and the extensive benefits derived from play in natural environments (Fjørtoft, 2004; Bird, 2007; Lester and Maudsley, 2007; Munoz, 2009), it is not clear whether physical activity in a natural setting provides additive benefits for psychological wellbeing in children and young people.

Wood et al. (2013a) compared the effects of cycling whist viewing either rural or urban scenes on self-esteem and mood in adolescents: physical activity alone improved self-esteem and mood via reductions in tension, but there were no differences in the change in self-esteem and mood as a result of viewing different environmental scenes. These findings are also supported by Duncan et al. (2014), who found that cycling whilst viewing a forest video provided no additive benefits for the mood of primary school children compared with cycling alone.

Several studies have also examined the effect of being directly exposed to differing environmental types. Reed et al. (2013) compared the effects of running in natural and urban environments and found that whilst the physical activity improved self-esteem, there were no differences in the improvements in self-esteem. These findings are supported by Wood et al. (2014a) who found no differences in the change in self-esteem between play on the playground and field; and Barton et al. (2014) who identified that a nature-based intervention was no more effective at increasing self-esteem than a playground-based intervention. Furthermore, Wood et al. (2014b) found that there were no differences in the change in self-esteem when orienteering in both a natural and built environment, even though the orienteering itself led to improvements in self-esteem.

This apparent lack of additional benefit could be attributed to the types of activities included in studies with children. Adult studies have primarily included walking activities which are of light intensity and enable participants to interact with the environment and with each other. Exercise in the studies with children primarily included running and cycling and might have been too intense for them to notice their surrounding environment (Wood et al., 2014b). This is evidenced by the work of Taylor and Kuo (2009) who examined the effect of walking in three different environments on the concentration of children with ADHD. The study found that walking in a park resulted in significantly better concentration than walking in a residential or downtown setting. The effect of walking in the park was as large as the deficit due to ADHD and the peak effect of medication. Thus, the natural environment may only provide additive benefits for psychological wellbeing at low exercise intensities. It might also have a clear role for children suffering from attention deficit disorders and perhaps those with mental ill-health. Furthermore, in order to benefit from green exercise, children and young people might need direct interaction with nature (Wood et al., 2014a, b), such as is received from forest school and outdoor adventure programmes.

Children's disconnections with nature

This lack of green exercise effect could also be attributed to children and young people's low levels of everyday interaction with nature. As a society we spend less time outdoors, both in working and leisure contexts. As a result, we are becoming increasingly disconnected from nature.

Connection to nature is described as the degree to which an individual includes nature as part of their identity (Schultz, 2002) and it includes an understanding of nature and everything it comprises, both good and bad (Nisbet et al., 2009). Connectedness to nature is also an important predictor of subjective wellbeing and ecological behaviour (Mayer and Frantz, 2004; Hine et al., 2008b). For example feelings of connectedness to nature reported after wilderness experiences range from the aesthetic appreciation of beautiful scenery and landscapes to a deep sense of belonging to the natural world. In this context nature connection has also been taken to include feelings of peacefulness and harmony, a sense of timelessness, creation of a sense of vulnerability which is humbling, learning a respect for nature and developing a sense of place (Russell 1999, 2001; Caulkins et al., 2006; Hine et al., 2009). However, not all children and young people have opportunities to interact with local urban nature, let alone experience more intense wilderness settings. The issues of contact and connection may also be interlinked, with increasing contact leading to increasing connection. It appears, however, that both connection to and interaction with nature are on the decline in affluent countries. Particular concerns have arisen about children's disconnection from nature and these have been brought to the fore by Richard Louv (2005): 'at the very moment that the bond is breaking between the young and the natural world, a growing body of research links our mental, physical, and spiritual health directly to our association with nature'.

The current generation of children and young people spends less time interacting with nature than previous generations and are thus increasingly confined to indoor and urban settings (Bird, 2007). The proportion of children playing out in natural spaces has dropped by some 75 per cent over the last 30 to 40 years, with only 10 per cent of young people having regular contact with nature compared with the 40 per cent of adults who did so 30–40 years ago (Natural England, 2009). A similar pattern has emerged in Australia suggesting this is an international problem. The average British child watches almost 2.5 hours of television per day (up 12 per cent since 2007) (OFCOM, 2011; Moss, 2012) and spends more than 20 hours a week online (IPPR, 2008). All of this is despite the proven positive effects that contact with nature has on physical and mental health, personal and social development, and even academic achievements and life pathways (RSPB, 2012).

The term *Nature Deficit Disorder* describes the human costs of disconnection and alienation from nature such as diminished use of the senses, attention difficulties and higher rates of emotional and physical illnesses (Louv, 2005). The term was originally adopted for children but more recently has also been used to refer also to adult disconnections. In order to benefit from having contact with nature, a connection and understanding of the natural world is likely to be required (Bratman et al., 2012). Thus, children and young people might not benefit from green exercise in the same way as adults as a result of their prior or existing lack of connection to the natural world (Reed et al., 2013; Barton et al., 2014; Wood et al., 2014a, b). The continuing loss of connection to nature could then result in policy makers and environmentalists of the future having a lack of understanding of nature and its value (Pyle, 1978; Bird, 2007; Bragg et al., 2012). Evidence suggests people who do not value and respect nature when they are young are less likely to see the importance of protecting the natural environment when older (Pyle, 1978; Bird, 2007; Bragg et al., 2012). The increasing disconnection from nature in children and young people could have important consequences for future generations and the natural environment itself.

Reconnecting children to nature

Given the concerns about children and young people's disconnections from nature and the body of evidence describing the beneficial effects of both contact with and play in natural environments, it is not surprising that a drive to reconnect children with the outdoors has been initiated (Natural England, 2009; RSPB, 2010; Moss, 2012). The importance of children's connection to and respect for nature has been recognised in the UN Convention on the Rights of the Child (UNCRC) which has been in force in the UK since 1992. Article 31 of the Convention states that 'education of the child shall be directed to ... the development of respect for the natural environment' (UNCRC 29.1e) and that children should 'engage in play' (UNCRC 31). Furthermore, the results of recent research suggests that environmental educators should provide time during their specific 'Environmental Education' programmes for children to experience nature, enabling them to bond with the natural world by just being in nature (Natural

England, 2009; RSPB, 2010; Moss, 2012). Additional research also suggests that the focus on learning in the core-subject areas may have drawn attention away from opportunities to form emotional connections to nature through free play (Natural England, 2009; RSPB, 2010; Moss, 2012).

In 2009, Natural England examined the changing relationship between childhood and nature across generations, the extent of children's disengagement from nature and then highlighted the need for remedial action. This was supported by the RSPB's Every Child Outdoors report (RSPB, 2010) which brought together research about the wide benefits to children of being connected to nature; and the National Trust's national Outdoor Nation debate (later published as Natural Childhood: Moss, 2012); and creation of 'Project Wild thing', all of which explored children's contemporary relationship with nature. In addition, the UK government's Natural Environment White Paper 2011 The natural choice: securing the value of nature, saw acknowledgement of the importance of enabling children to connect with natural environments and to learn about nature. It called for an assurance that every child would have opportunities to visit natural environments (Defra, 2011). In 2012 the RSPB acknowledged the need to establish a baseline of connection to nature levels in the UK to allow longitudinal comparisons to be made and to enable assessment of the effectiveness of nature re-connection programmes. Subsequently the RSPB has developed appropriate methodologies for connection to nature surveys in children, adults and teenagers (Bragg and Wood, 2015) and is currently conducting baseline surveys across the UK. Natural England, Defra and the Forestry Commission have also acknowledged the importance of measuring connection to nature in children by piloting it in their Monitor of Engagement with the Natural Environment (MENE) survey, comprising 45,000 interviews annually, and providing trend data for how people use the natural environment in England (Natural England, 2015).

Conclusions

Play in natural environments provides a number of important health and wellbeing benefits to children and young people including increased levels of physical activity and improved psychological health outcomes. However, young people are increasingly confined to indoor and urban environments and as a result are becoming disconnected from nature. In order to reconnect children and young people with nature they should be encouraged to engage with the natural environment from a young age and to participate in more outdoor exercise and play. This will encourage more frequent countryside visits throughout adulthood and access to the health and social capital benefits associated with regular contact with nature (Peacock et al., 2007; Pretty et al., 2015).

Chapter 6

Learning on the move

Green exercise for children and young people

Liz O'Brien, Bianca Ambrose-Oji, Sue Waite, Jennie Aronsson and Maria Clark

Introduction

Physical activity is a key component of green education in nature ranging from mild to moderate or vigorous kinds of exercise. Acknowledging the role that formal and informal green education can play in enabling and encouraging physical activity is also important. These approaches can help to reduce sedentary behaviours and have positive impacts on obesity, type 2 diabetes, and mental resilience (Department of Health, 2011b). Here we outline the concept of green education and explore connections with physical activity. We identify how this links to broader health and wellbeing and consider how green education fits into current education policy, and provide examples from the United Kingdom illustrating current approaches to practice and research with primary school age children (4–11 years) and young excluded people (14–25 years). We argue that green education can play an important role in improving children and young people's physical activity levels and has a strong impact on their broader wellbeing.

What is green education?

Our definition of green education (also called outdoor learning, learning outside the classroom, outdoor education, and learning in natural environments (LINE)) extends beyond learning about the natural environment and developing positive environmental attitudes. We understand it as a situated natural and cultural context for learning any subject or skill, which brings greater opportunities for people to trial different ways of being and learning than when indoors (Waite, 2013; Waite and Pratt, 2015). It is not only about children's school learning outside the classroom but includes informal learning opportunities for all ages. 'Green education seems to be a more holistic concept [than environmental or sustainable education] and can include learning about either a) nature or b) other subjects; but the key element is being outside' (Bragg et al., 2013). Recent research by Lin et al. (2014) suggests that the opportunities of being outside are unlikely to be sufficient and that orientation through education, for example, is a more significant predictor of future use of greenspaces than solely accessibility.

Kellert (2012) suggests that starting early helps to develop a positive desire to be in nature. Internationally, many early years' policies recognise the outdoor environment as important for children's development (Maynard and Waters, 2014). Green education is recognised as also providing significant personal, social and health outcomes (Lovell and Roe, 2009; Dillon and Dickie, 2012). It can also increase engagement and attainment in curricular subjects (Ofsted, 2008). This diversity of potential benefits is, however, shaped by the current educational context, particularly in nations that are pursuing a performativity agenda of standards (NEETF, 2000; Waite and Pleasants, 2012). Green education is consequently often harnessed to mainstream educational ends. This presents some challenges (Rea and Waite, 2012) for co-opting the wider benefits of this learning to the service of formal education that arguably has narrower aspirations and vision of what constitutes education for children and young people (Berliner, 2011). However, mainstreaming can offer a route to accessing the myriad benefits from learning in natural environments to a wider cohort (Bauman et al., 2012). For the majority of children in affluent countries, school represents a common denominator in their lives. Schooling can, therefore, address issues across different communities and socioeconomic groups, providing a 'universal' access that many other methods of intervention directed at childhood experience would struggle to achieve.

Although we focus particularly on the benefits for physical wellbeing, one of the strengths of outdoor learning is that it can address a number of aims simultaneously (Dillon and Dickie, 2012). As we shall see below, it may be both prudent and politic to foreground these multiple potential outcomes in order to encourage the use of natural environments for the achievement of physical health outcomes.

Research is beginning to unpick subtleties in what the contribution of different outdoor spaces might be, so that concepts such as 'green education' and 'the great outdoors' are being defined more precisely. Studies are distinguishing and subdividing into, for example: blue aquatic environments (White et al., 2010); wilderness experiences (Cordell et al., 2005); familiar local natural environments (Beames and Ross, 2010); different cultural, geographical and historical milieu (Stewart, 2008; Wattchow and Brown, 2011; Waite, 2013); managed parks and landscapes (Ward Thompson et al., 2012); school grounds (Malone and Tranter, 2003; Waite, 2013), woodland and forests (O'Brien, 2009); and therapeutic and school gardens (Sempik and Aldridge, 2006; Passy et al., 2010).

This more nuanced approach has resulted in greater variety and specificity of research studies, rapidly increasing the depth and breadth of the evidence base related to specific educational interventions in particular natural contexts. However, many of these studies are small scale and unpublished, and fail to build effectively on each other.

Elements that need to be considered in green education research and practice include the following questions:

- Purpose – what? why?
- Place – where?

- Pedagogy – how?
- People – who?

Waite (2014, 2015) suggests that 'minding these ps and qs' provides a structure whereby the situated characteristics of learning outdoors in natural environments can be made more visible. This can maximise their learning potential and provide an analytical framework. First, the teacher needs to consider what the educational purpose is in taking learning outside the classroom. If this is to engender discovery and creative learning in the children, then teachers may choose a place that will support that by locating the lesson within a novel context that is not weighted with prior expectations. Waite (2013) refers to this as a 'culturally light' place where new ways of being and thinking may be better supported than in a familiar context which is 'dense' with cultural norms. For example, a visit to local woodland may offer an exciting context for imaginative story construction, where teachers and children can play with different ideas and narratives. In such a case, the pedagogy employed is likely to be facilitative rather than directive and follow children's lines of interest. The people involved in learning may include peers since group work encourages children to explore different ideas rather than seek the answer that they think the teacher wants (Mercer et al., 1999).

In another lesson the focus may be on developing knowledge of geographical and cultural features of the landscape; here the place is likely to be visited repeatedly to build understanding of it and a relationship with it. For example, Beames and Ross (2010) have worked with schools in Scotland on 'Outdoor Journeys' that develop cultural familiarity with places to stimulate sustained project-based learning. This pedagogical approach may require expert knowledge of the area, possibly including other adults who can provide historical details about the culture that is embedded in the place. In Ireland the 'Heritage in Schools Expert scheme' encourages this by inviting people who are expert in heritage to support school learning.

If the teaching aim is to stimulate different sorts of physical activity, open beaches may encourage more cardiovascular activity through running, while places with uneven terrain such as wooded areas may encourage finer body control (Fjørtoft, 2004). Aronsson et al. (2014) found that lower levels of children's moderate to vigorous physical activity were associated with school grounds compared to woodland. People supporting this kind of learning may also find that modelling vigorous movement is an effective pedagogical strategy.

Thus contexts for green educational endeavour are becoming more refined and there is greater attention to the nature of pedagogy within these spaces and its alignment with educational or health and wellbeing purposes. Innovative strategies may be necessary to address growing concerns around health and wellbeing and to capitalise on increasing evidence of the benefits of green education for health.

Evidencing the links between green spaces and behaviour

The evidence suggests that the relationships and the kind of benefits linked to physical activity in natural environments varies by age, gender, ethnicity, socioeconomic status and degrees of social cohesion (Lachowycz et al., 2012; de Vries et al., 2013; Dinnie et al., 2013). This emphasises our argument that research and practice need to understand the responses of people, i.e. children and young people with different social and cultural characteristics, within the matrix of place, pedagogy and learning purpose. The evidence base covering the links between physical activity and greenspace for children and young people, particularly for those from more disadvantaged backgrounds, is relatively small. What research there is for children and young people shows: children are more likely to engage in moderate to vigorous levels of exercise when spending time with friends outdoors (Pearce et al., 2014); over half of moderate to vigorous activity in children occurs in urban greenspace and mostly at weekends (Lachowycz et al., 2012); and young people gain social and mental health benefits from recreation in particular urban green settings (Moore et al., 2014).

It is not just the presence of green (e.g. parks, woods) and blue (e.g. streams, lakes, ponds) outdoor spaces which is important to leveraging specific impacts. The planning and design of greenspaces is important and has been shown to change usage patterns and behaviours according to age and other socio-demographic factors (Ward Thompson et al., 2008 and 2013). People's engagement and use of the environment depends on the types and quality of the greenspace, how close it is to them, and issues such as ease of access and site infrastructure provision. It also depends on factors such as the availability of organised and informal activities introducing people to specific sites and different kinds of ecosystems and habitats (Lin et al., 2014). Education, training and learning activities in the outdoors can mediate all these functions (Children and Nature Network, 2012). For younger age groups this encompasses activities such as adventure play e.g. den building, pond dipping, tree climbing, and for young people activities such as group and individual sports, or environmental science experimentation, and importantly includes all curriculum learning that takes place outside the classroom. Such organised and informal learning can counter the 'cotton wool kids' trend (O'Connor and Brown, 2013), and encourage active exercise, general fitness as well as bone and muscle strengthening, improving gross and fine motor skills, and motor coordination: patterns of activity that are potentially carried forward throughout life.

Current education policy

While factors at the level of practice need to be kept in mind, learning approaches and opportunities for the integration of outdoor activity are shaped and constrained by the wider educational policy context. In Scandinavian countries outdoor culture permeates society, and there is a greater willingness to embrace broader concepts of education as developing the whole person (bildung) (Bentsen and Jensen, 2012). Consequently, outdoor learning is much better established in Scandinavian education policies (Bentsen, 2013). Bildung has more in common with English early years educational and care provision that encourages a whole child perspective, so in England outdoor learning is better integrated in the early years than at later stages of education (Waite, 2010). As Waite (2010) notes, the decline of children's opportunities to learn outdoors has been influenced by policies encouraging performativity and a narrowing of curriculum aims that high stakes testing regimes tend to produce (Berliner, 2011). In Denmark, the government has recently funded a large Continuing Professional Development programme to support the spread of udeskole, where children learn curricular subjects outside the classroom: the physical, cognitive and social benefits arising from this practice are being examined by a complementary research project (Mygind, 2013).

Existing research has shown the value of outdoor learning for cognitive attainment (National Environmental Education and Training Foundation, 2000; Dillon and Dickie, 2012;) and the associated value of physical activity for academic attainment by helping to change attitudes and academic behaviours such as concentration and attention (CDC, 2010). The new curriculum in England, introduced from September 2014 (Department for Education, 2013), although somewhat prescriptive in content, has responded to this evidence, and makes reference to the importance of experiential learning in contexts other than the classroom. Furthermore, educational policies in Scotland, Wales and Ireland have advocated outdoor learning, reflecting a global popular movement that supports reconnection of children with nature (Louv, 2008; Moss, 2012; Council for Learning Outside the Classroom) alongside concern with sedentary lifestyles and childhood obesity (Marmot, 2010). Natural Connections is a recent example of a project funded by Natural England, Department for Environment and Rural Affairs (DEFRA) and English Heritage, that responds to this evidence base and the policy imperatives outlined in the English government's Natural Environment White Paper — The Natural Choice: Securing the Value of Nature (HM Government, 2011). The project seeks to embed learning in outdoor and natural contexts across the curriculum in primary and secondary phases.

In Britain in the past, children with special educational needs have benefitted from additional funding and the development of alternative curricula, and pedagogical approaches such as Forest Schools, that have used green education as an effective approach to engage these groups with learning. Less affected by high stakes testing, there was less pressure on teachers to achieve high academic scores, and greater freedom to experiment with these pupil groups. However, contemporary financial pressures mean that there are now other school priorities for budget allocation. Schools in areas of high multiple deprivation or with high numbers of children with special educational needs may struggle to reach the performance standards set, and may now be less willing to widen and enrich the curriculum offer at the risk of failing to meet targets for 'what counts'. In such circumstances it is the availability of funding and performative demands of policy, rather than the appropriateness of the green education approach, that often dictates pedagogy and outcomes. However, schools with high levels of eligible students, and which recognise the benefits accruing from green education, may choose to use their pupil premium (additional funding given to publicly funded schools in England to raise the attainment of disadvantaged pupils) creatively to ensure that children who would not otherwise access nature have the opportunity to do so.

Citizenship and personal social and health education (PSHE) is another major strand of outdoor learning policy and practice. Since the early days of the outdoor education movement, outdoor and adventurous activity has been advocated as a means to developing this fundamental learning in young people (Neill, 2003); although acquisition and transferability of personal and social skills from the particular learning situation is contested by place-based scholars such as Brookes, (2007). Nevertheless, examples of this philosophy being carried forward are the many social action projects carried out in outdoor contexts, e.g. creating community gardens within the National Citizen Service, an English government initiative to build a bigger and stronger society (Natcen, 2013).

Cross government policy aimed at older children and young people aged 13–19 includes 'Positive for Youth'. The policy recognises that some young people (about 6 per cent) experience complex and multiple needs including NEET (Not in Employment, Education or Training) status, having low educational attainment and difficult behaviours such as misusing substances (Cabinet Office and Department for Education, 2010). The policy vision focuses on the development of supportive relationships, the encouragement of strong ambitions and the provision of good opportunities as crucial aspects for preparing young people for work and adult life. There is potential for green education to contribute to this policy agenda by providing some good opportunities that can help prepare young people for work.

Opportunities for green education in lifelong and lifewide learning

This section provides examples of learning projects incorporating physical activity in natural contexts. Using the 'ps and qs' scheme (Purpose, Place, Pedagogy, People) as our framework, we describe each of the examples and explain the impacts on levels of participants' physical activity. The 'Place' in each of the examples is woodland, and the 'People' cover two specific age groups, i.e. primary school children aged 4–11 years; and young people aged 14–25 years. The latter group includes vulnerable and disadvantaged learners.

Woodland Health for Youth (WHY): an evaluation of physical health benefits derived from learning outside the classroom in natural environments (LINE) for school-age children

In spring 2014 research was conducted evaluating the health benefits of green education, called Learning In Natural Environments (LINE). The Woodland Health for Youth (WHY) project was a partnership between Plymouth City

Council (Stepping Stones to Nature, 2012), Plymouth University (School of Nursing and Midwifery and the Institute of Education), Plymouth Community Healthcare, Good from Woods and one of the local schools taking part in the Natural Connections project and offering LINE to their pupils. The aim of the evaluation was to measure the physical health benefits of LINE and assess the contribution of WHY to reducing the incidence of childhood obesity, as well as promoting better partnership working between health and education services (Marmot, 2010). The study explored the potential for outdoor learning as a framework for 'whole school health promotion' (Langford et al., 2014), appointing a nurse researcher for this initiative at the school.

An interdisciplinary action research design appropriate for change management in a clinical practice setting was chosen, based on a recursive helix of planning, acting, observing and reflecting (Robinson, 2011). A reflective log was kept throughout the project, which included observations, discussions, thoughts and any ideas that evolved as the project progressed. These emergent reflections fed into the research cycle and informed the process.

Children undertook lessons across a range of curriculum subjects within their local woodland with the purpose of stimulating their engagement in learning. The pedagogy employed encouraged active experiential learning. Ten children in a Year 2 class participated in the research, selected through a 'first-come first-served' based consent process, reflecting mixed gender and attainment within the sample. Quantitative data on physical activity was collected using accelerometers attached to each child's wrist of choice to measure indoor and outdoor activity throughout the school day. Accelerometry is an established technique translating detection of movement into physical activity levels (Cooper et al., 2010; Kim et al., 2012). The children wore the monitors for the entire school day, but not when they went home. Comparison with the school timetable allowed data to be segregated into indoor and outdoor lessons and break times. In addition to the accelerometers, children's height and weight were measured and their body mass index (BMI) was calculated. The measurements were compared to measurements done by the school nursing service two years earlier, in Reception year, as part of the National Child Measurement Programme (National Child Measurement Programme, 2013).

Figure 6.1 shows the proportion of time spent in moderate to vigorous physical activity in each context. Statistical analysis of the physical activity levels obtained through accelerometers demonstrated that children were significantly more active during LINE sessions than during indoor lessons (17.0% ± 6.7 SD in LINE sessions, 6.2% ± 4.3 in indoor lessons, p=0.000). They were particularly active when LINE was held in woodland (19.0% ± 7.1), rather than in the green school grounds (13.7% ± 4.8 in school ground LINE, p=0.01).

The woodland offers a larger and less familiar space to move around in, with ample opportunities to engage in a wide range of activities. Passy and Waite (2011) identify multiple benefits to woodland LINE including greater freedom, wilder and more natural space, child-led learning, negotiated boundaries, created activities and managed risk.

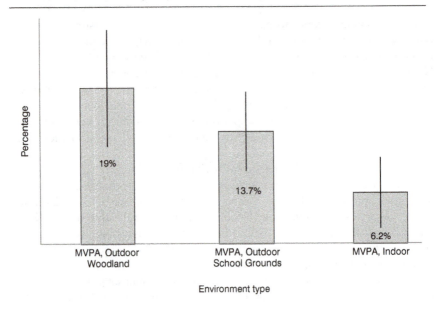

Figure 6.1 Levels of moderate to vigorous physical activity (MVPA) in different school environments (Aronsson et al, 2014)

While national and local data demonstrate an increase in childhood obesity year-on-year (Public Health, Plymouth City Council, 2013), the results of this small-scale study contradict this trend; the majority of children had lowered their BMI since Reception year measurements. In Year 2, eight out of ten children had a healthy BMI at the time of measurement while two were classified as overweight; none of the children were underweight or obese. A recent systematic review by Langford et al. (2014) highlights the link between physical activity interventions and BMI reduction. Although childhood obesity is complex with many factors influencing children's BMI, the WHY project suggests that physical activity through LINE may be a contributing factor to reversing the negative trend generally seen in children's BMI levels. Furthermore, LINE may offer a more equitable and consistent way of increasing overall physical activity levels compared to targeted interventions or increases in break time, by avoiding stigmatisation of overweight children or compounding sedentary patterns in free play.

Observational data also indicates that children engage in a range of different activities during LINE, so developing a multitude of skills in addition to curricular learning, such as gross and fine motor skills, risk-taking behaviour and safe practice, creative skills, social skills and building confidence and self-efficacy. Additionally, children's body language mirrored the joy these activities and the outdoor environment provided. Spontaneous comments made by the children demonstrate that some of the children enjoy LINE and spending time in the woodlands, linking LINE to their social, emotional and physical sense of wellbeing:

'This is fun!' (girl looking for insects on a tree).

'I love nature' (boy in the woodland).

'I can feel the sun in my face and the fresh air' (girl in the woodland).

The WHY evaluation associated school-based initiatives and access to greenspace with increased physical activity levels; suggesting possible positive long-term health outcomes. To be effective, sustainable and equitable, LINE needs to become a regular feature of schooling, perhaps even enshrined in the national curriculum, in order to give all children, regardless of socioeconomic background, equal opportunity to access natural environments and to enjoy the multiple benefits that come with this.

Importantly green education such as LINE also provides a much wider range of benefits for children and young people. The concept of lifewide learning is outlined by Jackson (2014) as learning that takes place across the different roles and spaces people inhabit; at work, home, in education, in the hobbies and interests people pursue. This concept is illustrated in some of the examples below.

Physical activity through training and volunteering programmes for excluded 14–25 year olds

Hill Holt Wood (HHW) is a social enterprise that provides green education opportunities for pupils excluded from school. HHW works with Lincolnshire County Council as part of a programme called 'Solutions 4' involving young men excluded from mainstream education. A member of the HHW Board said 'it's impossible to underestimate the brutalising effects of where most of these kids live' (O'Brien, 2005a, b). One of the venues for 'Solutions 4' pupils is HHW, a small 14-hectare wood: they can choose to attend if they are interested in woodlands, conservation and outdoor working.

One study explored the activities of HHW (O'Brien, 2005a, b). Since then the wood has developed further to provide a wide range of opportunities for health, education and architectural design in woodlands (HHW undated). The pedagogical approach at HHW is to provide a strong ethos giving support and structure for the boys. The tasks are changed and adapted so that their attention span can be managed, and they can produce artefacts, such as wooden spoons, quickly. The focus is on progressing and providing learning opportunities that are appropriate for the boys when mainstream schooling has not worked. The young men participate in conservation, construction, tourism as well as undertake basic English, ICT (information and communication technologies) and Maths. They are also encouraged to include and bring their parents and carers to the wood at weekends and to plant their own tree 'so whatever happens… they can always come back to HHW; and because it's a community woodland, they always can' (HHW staff member). The physical elements of the approach can play an important role in helping to calm the young men. One of the teaching staff talked about the boys and the woodland environment and said 'they were coming away from something, coming into something completely different, the fresh air was tiring them and the physicality of the work'.

Project Scotland (PS, 2014) is a volunteer placement programme for young people aged 16–30 years classified as NEET. They receive a subsistence allowance for undertaking a minimum of 30 hours of activity per week, for between three and twelve months. A Project Scotland programme was set up by Forestry Commission Scotland (FCS) in Galloway Forest for young men aged 16–25 years, drawn from areas with few employment opportunities to undertake practical conservation volunteering (O'Brien et al., 2010, 2011). Galloway Forest is a large wooded area in southern Scotland that includes moorland, hills and lochs. The aim of the programme was to give the young men an opportunity to learn new skills, gain confidence, work as part of a team and potentially move into further education or employment. A research project on conservation volunteering included the FCS programme, with data being gathered through interviews and questionnaires (O'Brien et al., 2011).

Most of the young men were aged 16 and 17; some experienced behavioural and emotional difficulties as well as substance abuse. One young man said if it were not for Project Scotland: 'we'd all be sitting at home drinking Export [a brand of lager] and on the laptop'. Getting out of the house, being outdoors and doing something positive were all considered important by the young men (O'Brien et al., 2011). The activities they undertook included brashing, ditching, removing vegetation, they gained training in chainsaw and strimmer use, fencing and pesticide application. The work was often physically active; one young man noted 'you sleep better' when active. Activities including mountain biking, football and barbeques were also organised for the young men outside of the volunteering activity as part of celebrations providing further opportunities for the young men to be physically active.

Phoenix Futures (PF, undated) runs a 'recovery through nature' programme which aims to aid people's recovery through undertaking tasks in nature. 'As an organisation, what's important to us is not the actual activity itself or the task at hand, it's about taking part... we provide them with the skills to plan out a task, delegate tasks, take on responsibilities, delegate responsibilities, so it encourages them to take ownership of the whole programme' (PF representative). As part of a wider study, on Forestry Commission Scotland's engagement with communities, an interview was undertaken with a representative from PF (Lawrence et al., 2014). PF won a contract from FCS to deliver a skills programme for unemployed 16–25-year-olds in Glasgow. The work is undertaken on FCS-managed forest land or other publicly owned land. The young people are taught forestry skills which include chainsaw training, scrub cutting, pruning and landscaping. They are often socially excluded, isolated and using drugs and alcohol. The work the young people undertake involves a range of physical activity from mild to very active. The physical activity, physical experience, gaining improvements in gross and fine motor skills and co-ordination of movement are important aspects of the training the young people receive (Hall, 2004).

Supported by Natural England's 'Access to Nature' programme, 'Into the Woods' was launched in September 2011. Based in Bristol it specialises in working with young adults and adults from vulnerable backgrounds. Discussions with project leaders as part of a short research project looking at mindfulness-based approaches to using the outdoors (Ambrose-Oji, 2013), explained that the purpose of the green education programme is to deliver positive physical and mental health benefits to participants with learning difficulties, disabilities or are mental health service users through physical activity in woodland settings. This group of people do not normally tend to access natural environments, either because they find these surroundings unfamiliar and frightening or because transport or physical access may be difficult. The pedagogic approach employed by the project is an adapted form of 'Forest School'. Participants are encouraged to explore the natural world through all of their senses, using environmental art, bush craft and developing traditional woodland working techniques.

For those young adults with capacity, traditional forestry and woodland skills training involves coppicing and hedge laying, but trainees are also introduced to activities such as fire lighting, tool care and health and safety management. For participants with particularly severe learning disabilities, the education and training is focused on developing self-confidence and key life skills through 'taking notice', developing awareness of the woodland environment and personal connections with it.

The project leaders reported an evaluation of the outcomes using indicators developed within the Silvanus Trust (undated) and Plymouth University 'Good from Woods' project showed that taking participants to new and challenging environments increased physical and emotional engagement with the environment, and encouraged new ways of exercising. It also broadens participant expectations of the kinds of physical activity they can take part in, as well as outdoor employment and volunteering opportunities they might apply for.

Discussion

We have outlined the importance of physical activity as a critical component of green education. This has an impact not only on children and young people's physical health but also on their mental resilience and wellbeing, self-esteem and social connections. The 'WHY' research project provides an innovative example of the education, environment and health sectors working together to research the levels of physical activity that can occur in green education compared to a traditional school day. This type of approach has potential for wider impact if adopted as part of whole school health promotion. The examples of 14–25 year olds all involve young people with major problems who are often facing exclusion and isolation. Green education is shown to be particularly effective for some of these young people due to the atmosphere of the environment which can be calming, therapeutic and restorative, especially for those with anger management and behavioural problems. Much satisfaction can be gained by individuals connecting with nature and for some this can be a whole new experience. Changes in attitudes and behaviour occur and may be promoted through improved physical self-image and positive physical exercise. These behaviours can potentially last beyond the green education experience into adult life and lifewide learning (Pretty et al., 2009; Jackson, 2014).

Green design and planning

There is potential for the environment and education sectors, with support and input from the health sector, to start working more closely together to encourage the design and creation of greenspace infrastructure in:

i   any new build school, nursery, college and university development
ii existing education establishments which provide opportunities to retrofit green infrastructure/space.

Such approaches are starting in collaborations between the health and environment sectors such as the NHS (National Health Service) Forest in England and Wales and in the NHS Greenspace demonstration project in Scotland (O'Brien, 2014). Both of these programmes create greenspace in new or existing health care settings from hospitals to doctors' surgeries. In other examples, education establishments will be encouraged to utilise these and other nearby greenspaces for green education. Forestry Commission Scotland for example, provides information on public forest learning sites close to schools that can be used for programmes such as Forest School (FCS, 2009). Natural Connections has had significant impact promoting the educational use of schools' local natural environments, including beaches, their grounds and nearby parks and woodland.

Perhaps one of the most persuasive aspects about green education is research that shows that even outside of formal education, nature is a learning resource that promotes resilience in young people positively affecting their future life course. Merchant et al.'s (2013) study of young people in low-skilled jobs in the southwest of England unexpectedly found that many drew on nature as a positive factor in their lives. Other research examining social and economic aspirations of young people living in or near a national park (Merchant et al., 2013) demonstrated how strongly they valued the natural environment, and how significant it was to their life choices, influencing their future occupational training and extending the time they remained within their local community.

The Monitor Engagement with the Natural Environment (MENE) survey reports on visits with children to nature by adults from 2009–2012 (Natural England, 2012) in England. It found that 37 per cent of visits with children were within 1 mile of home with parks in a town or city being the most visited nature spaces (Natural England, 2012). Motivations to visit nature for those with children were to entertain and play with them; 40 per cent of visits to nature with children involved play and 59 per cent walking. Children that canvas for time in natural environments may also be a force to green educate their parents.

The RSPB report Every Child Outdoors (2010) concluded that 'there is strong evidence to show that by the time children leave secondary school, their attitude to exercise is highly predictive of whether they will be physically active as adults. The strongest relationship is with the quality of exercise they have experienced, as opposed to the quantity of exercise. Nature is a major motivating factor for exercise'.

Encouraging these behaviours relies on greenspace design that provides children and young people with welcoming, nearby access and environments that stimulate their need to explore and safely challenges them (NICE, 2008). A focus on greenspace and formal learning approaches such as those outlined in this chapter, when combined with improvements to the quality, facilities and visual welcome of existing greenspace for children and young people, can consequently encourage greenspace access as part of everyday living and family life for lifewide learning. The challenge is for policy makers, planners and practitioners to recognise the value of greenspaces in this context, and find the means to protect, maintain and improve public and other accessible greenspace during a period of global and national economic austerity (Heritage Lottery Fund, 2014).

Wider benefits than physical activity

This chapter focused on the importance of green education in encouraging and enabling physical activity, but we emphasise that much wider benefits and opportunities are provided for children and young people. For example, the young men at Galloway Forest talked about sensory experiences that were an important part of the whole physical experience. They enjoyed seeing wildlife and wanted to take care of it, appreciated the views of nature, felt a sense of freedom 'yeah it's got me, got in my veins' (Young man, Project Scotland, Galloway), gained a sense of place and felt more at ease. Green education can be a particularly important approach for those who face specific issues, such as attention deficit hyperactivity disorder (Faber Taylor and Kuo, 2011), anger, behavioural and emotional difficulties and kinaesthetic learners who learn by doing (O'Brien and Murray, 2007). Understanding this wide range of benefits and their association with different natural contexts can enable green educators to target green education appropriately for different audiences and sectors.

Cross-sector partnerships

Partnership working is essential to the success of planning, design, governance and the delivery of green education whether formal or informal. Our examples show partnerships across the environment and education sectors, and, more infrequently, with the health sector. Some of the barriers to partnership working that the projects overcame included differing objectives and requirements for reporting, siloed working and thinking, diverse professional cultures and a lack of a common language or understanding between sectors, inequality of input and the time needed to develop partnerships. It can be important to consider different types of partnership working. For example, strategic partnerships focus on high impact relationships involving integration into governance and decision-making processes. Policy delivery partnerships aim at a specific policy target; while operational partnerships focus on organising specific practical programmes and projects (Ambrose-Oji et al., 2010). There can also be partnerships concentrating on networking in which there is sharing of information, communication and contacts (Ambrose-Oji et al., 2010). To date, the majority of green education projects have been operational projects and programmes that are time limited. Without strategic networking, lessons are not necessarily being learnt across these projects and scaling them up remains difficult. This highlights the importance of the strategic partnerships explored within the Natural Connections project to raise the profile and impact of green education not only as an approach to learning but an effective policy approach to tackling the 'physical inactivity epidemic' (All Party Commission on Physical Inactivity, 2014).

With recent health and social care reforms in England decentralising responsibility for public health back to Local Authorities there are new opportunities to support schools in promoting healthy schools and pupils (Buck and Gregory, 2013). Green education approaches offer an effective approach to achieve this by incorporating more physical activity into the curriculum. Indeed, the link between pedagogy, people and place is strengthened with such devolution since Local Authorities are also responsible for significant areas of public parks and other open spaces, and often work in partnership with others from the environment sector such as the Forestry Commission in planning the use of other public land (Tighe et al., 2013). Agreements can also be reached with private sector landowners for green education to take place on their land (Murray and O'Brien, 2005).

Interventions encouraging green education

The examples provided in this chapter illustrate a range of different types of interventions that enable and encourage green education. Evidence suggests that interventions targeting the wider social environment of individuals can also be important (Morris et al., 2012; O'Brien and Morris, 2013). For example, families, community structures and social networks can play a significant role in bringing about sustained change. Interventions that involve participants in the design of the intervention can also ensure the needs of those targeted are met (Morris et al., 2012).

The limitations of project-delivered interventions is that they tend to be short term lasting two to four years. Progress made by project leaders can, therefore, be restricted. This can be exacerbated where project-based working sees project leaders leaving before the end of the intervention to secure continuing employment in new posts. Accessing further funding to extend a successful intervention is also difficult. Funding bodies tend to prefer new projects to be 'innovative' and differing from previous ones, even if extending a funding scheme might extend reach, embed success and increase impact.

Research gaps

There has been research that has explored physical activity levels and the wider benefits of green education. However, this evidence base remains limited in crucial ways including many diverse and dispersed small-scale studies involving small numbers of participants with cross-sectional rather than longitudinal timescales that limit assessment of the complex relationships and interactions between physical, social and educational benefits over time. Evaluations of green education interventions are often restricted by a lack of baseline data or by the small scale of funds allocated as the majority of the funding often goes on delivery of the intervention. The WHY study suggests further research on physical activity on a larger scale and over a longer period, with appropriate use of accelerometers would be useful. But this needs to be coupled with exploration of the leadership role in promoting physical activity, enabling robust evidence to be gathered to inform partnership approaches to whole school health promotion. The general need remains for research with greater specificity of 'purpose, people, place, and pedagogy' in order to provide better understanding and assessment of the most effective approaches for specific groups of children and young people.

Conclusions

As Britain and other countries integrate a public health focus across policies of all kinds, it seems there has never been a better time to embed green education as a cross-sectoral approach to improving physical activity levels amongst children and young people. As this chapter demonstrates in formal learning, for example, this means moving from a focus in schools that is mainly on sports, towards integration of outdoor learning across the curricula. Better recognition of the evidence that outdoor spaces are not equal, that different habitats and natural settings afford different opportunities for physical exercise and facilitate different learning outcomes, should provide planners, designers and practitioners in the environmental, land management, public, private and civil society sectors with strategies for 'designing in' opportunities for physical and restorative activity. Our examples have demonstrated that woodlands provide a 'culturally light', and particularly flexible and valuable space for the physical and mental health benefits offered by green education.

We have shown how green education crosses the formal/informal education divide acting as an effective vehicle to support a lifelong/lifewide concept of learning and personal development. There is often complementarity between mainstreaming green education and supporting informal lifewide learning.

The 'pester power' of children may persuade parents and carers to visit natural settings young people have been exposed to as a setting for green education. This can bring play, learning and exercise into other parts of family life, promoting beneficial behaviours across the generations.

The chapter also demonstrates the potential of green education to deliver outcomes related to social justice and health inequalities. Many green education initiatives are targeted at disadvantaged members of society who often suffer with poorer life chances and poorer health status but may feel stigmatised by special treatment. The chapter has also shown the potential of mainstreaming green education approaches to ensure a more universal access to outdoor settings and the benefits derived from them to all school children.

Policy embedded support that maintains sight of 'purpose, people, place and pedagogy' (Waite, 2014) and a broad interpretation of green education as 'learning on the move', could secure the widest set of benefits from outdoor physical activity in the years to come.

Chapter 7

The health benefits of blue exercise in the UK

Mathew P. White, Sarah Bell, Lewis R. Elliott, Rebecca Jenkin, Benedict W. Wheeler and Michael H. Depledge

What do we mean by blue exercise?

We use the term 'Blue Exercise' to refer to physical activity undertaken in and around outdoor 'natural' aquatic environments such as lakes, rivers, canals and the coast (Depledge and Bird, 2009). These activities could involve being in the water (e.g. outdoor swimming/diving), on the water (e.g. sailing/canoeing), or simply by the water (e.g. walking along a canal tow-path). Given its popularity we also include recreational angling as a form of blue exercise. Although angling may seem to be associated with very little physical activity, energy expenditure estimates are similar to those for walking at a slow to moderate pace (Ainsworth et al., 2011). We do not, however, include swimming in man-made swimming pools, despite the fact that it is one of the most popular physical activities in the country with 13 per cent of men and 15 per cent of women reporting having been swimming within the past month (Stamatakis and Chaudhury, 2008). Although the motivations behind, and experiences of, such swimming are of interest and may promote positive outcomes (Barton et al., 2012) they are beyond the scope of the current chapter. Rather, consistent with the other chapters in this volume (as well as related articles, e.g. Pretty et al., 2005; Gladwell et al., 2013), our focus is on outdoor activities in natural, and in this case aquatic, environments.

We begin with a brief history of blue exercise in the UK, and in particular how environments often considered as hostile (especially the coast) came to be seen as places for leisure, recreation and physical activity. Then we consider recent data on blue exercise participation in the UK. This section briefly reviews data from the Health Survey for England (HSE) and the Watersports and Leisure Participation Survey (WLPS) before presenting novel analysis on data relating to blue exercise in Natural England's Monitor of Engagement with the Natural Environment (MENE) survey. The main questions explored in this section are what activities are undertaken, where and by whom? The third main section considers more epidemiological analysis looking at general levels of physical activity in relation to people's home proximity to blue space. The main questions here relate to whether living near blue spaces encourages blue exercise and in turn whether there is evidence that this may ultimately benefit health. The final section provides a short discussion on blue exercise and children. Much of the currently available data is focused on adults and yet there may be important opportunities for children to engage in blue exercise that are either not currently being researched and/or taken up. We conclude with some final thoughts about the role of blue exercise in the wider green exercise agenda.

A brief history of blue exercise in the UK

The coast has seen various shifts in cultural interpretation over time, from its enjoyment amongst the Ancient Greeks and Romans as a place of pleasure and beauty, its avoidance throughout The Middle Ages as a hostile and untamed place (perhaps in part driven by the Judeo-Christian biblical 'Deluge' narrative), and its gradual reintegration into societal activities from the 1700s onwards. This reintegration largely stemmed from: (a) the notion of the 'Sublime' and its influence on Romanticism; and (b) a desire for more hygienic, 'exclusive' alternatives to public bathing houses which had grown in popularity across society throughout the 1600s (Lenček and Bosker, 1998).

Ideas of the Sublime played a particular role in reshaping attitudes towards nature in the 1700s, as depicted in philosopher Edmund Burke's description of the sea as "a sort of delightful horror, a sort of tranquillity tinged with terror" (written in his 1757 treatise 'On the Sublime and Beautiful', cited by Lenček and Bosker, 1998: 550). These ideas captured the imagination of an influential Romantic literary, artistic and musical movement of the 1800s. Poets such as Wordsworth, Byron and Shelley depicted *unspoilt* nature (including coastal environments) as the gateway to self-knowledge and, through their poetry, inspired ideas about how best to experience nature in order to feel a sense of emotional release and spiritual renewal (Lenček and Bosker, 1998).

This coincided with a physician-led movement towards medicinal sea bathing, primarily amongst the so-called wealthier classes. The combination of *pure* sea air and the shock of cold salt water immersion were lauded by physicians as a cure for a growing list of actual and perceived illnesses of the time. In 1796, the Royal Sea Bathing Infirmary was opened in Margate as a "world pioneer for marine hospitals" (Fox and Lloyd, 1938), followed by Scarborough's Royal Northern Sea Bathing Infirmary in 1812. Bathing was carried out from a bathing machine platform with the assistance of a physician, early in the morning to prevent the risk of skin coloration (which was at the time associated with the 'labour classes'). This was followed by an invigorating stroll or horse ride along the beach in order to maximise sea air intake, which was believed to contain a higher concentration of oxygen than that inland. As this practice became increasingly popular, promenades were built to segregate bathers from fishermen and coastal workers, bathing attire was introduced, and areas were zoned to separate male and female bathing (Lenček and Bosker, 1998).

During the 1830s, an influential surgeon in Manchester, John Robertson, lamented the exclusivity of sea bathing, highlighting it as "the prerogative of the rich" (Fox and Lloyd, 1938). He facilitated the establishment of coastal convalescent homes for "crowded and debilitated factory workers" and the "feeble and disabled" who, he argued, "deserved and required, as much as the opulent, the means of recovery" provided by coastal settings (1938: 37). The increasing popularity of sea bathing by the mid-1800s, together with a growing awareness of alternative beach activities following steam-fuelled excursions abroad, broadened the focus of time spent at the coast beyond purely medicinal forms of sea bathing to include recreational swimming and pleasure. With further improvements to the railway networks and increasing leisure time (resulting from the 1871 Bank Holiday Act), the beach experience was gradually opened up to the 'middle' classes seeking to escape the crowded, polluted cities resulting from the Industrial Revolution (Lenček and Bosker, 1998).

The major shift towards the democratisation of the coast, however, occurred after World War I, when the motor engine created new opportunities for coastal access (enabling cheaper coach and rail travel, and a steady increase in car ownership). This contributed to the growth of informal temporary accommodation and holiday camps between the traditional guesthouse resorts established during the Victorian and Edwardian periods (Walton, 2000). These aimed to "set free the less moneyed public from the tyranny of furnished rooms" (Fox and Lloyd, 1938).

A post-World War I attitude reduced the formality of coastal activities during the inter-war period, with separate bathing abandoned in favour of families bathing together. Sunbathing became the norm as tanning was seen to reflect the luxury of leisure time and, therefore, no longer associated with the working classes. Many of those involved in the war saw the potential for freedom at the coast; "by immersing themselves in the sea, people could wash away the memories, the guilt and the pain; by basking in the sun, bake themselves back to health and vitality" (Lenček and Bosker, 1998: 201). Coinciding with the open air movement and the desire to stem the spread of tuberculosis, this inter-war period was characterised by outdoor pursuits, sports and entertainment (Walton, 2000). This was reflected in the building of new seaside features such as putting greens, bowling greens, cricket pitches, dance halls and art-deco cinemas. Such coastal resorts were particularly important during the 1930s, when the Great Depression restricted opportunities for holidays abroad.

The popularity of the UK coast continued until after World War II, although increasing affluence, paid holidays and car ownership sent many people further afield within the UK, looking to get away from the masses, the sprawling caravan parks and tired-looking pre-war resorts. A wave of seaside retirement to these pre-war resorts in the 1960s also led to growing tensions between residents craving the peace of the coast, and urban tourists looking for affordable coastal entertainment closer to home (Walton, 2000). With the rise in affordable air travel and the prevalence of overseas package holidays, the 1970s and 1980s saw a significant drop in domestic seaside holidays and coastal investment. This was compounded by increasing environmental concern about the impact of years of untreated coastal sewage disposal on British sea water quality. As a result, many

UK seaside resorts fell into decline, with a loss of fashionable identity and the legacy of what Paul Theroux termed 'seaside suburbia' (Walton, 2000).

Blue exercise in the UK today

What blue exercise is currently undertaken, by whom and how often? There are three major datasets which can be used to explore these questions. The first is the Health Survey for England (HSE). Over several years this survey has included questions on a large range of physical activities that people have engaged in, even just once, in the last four weeks. Reviewing data from several waves and including some 60,934 adults over 16 years, Stamatakis and Chaudhury (2008) report very low frequencies of a range of blue exercise activities for both men and women: sailing (male = 0.3 per cent; female = 0.1 per cent), rowing (male = 0.2 per cent; female = 0.1 per cent), canoeing (male = 0.2 per cent; female = 0.1 per cent), surfing (male = 0.1 per cent; female = <0.1 per cent), wind-surfing (male = 0.1 per cent; female = <0.1 per cent) and scuba-diving (male = 0.1 per cent; female = 0.1 per cent). Although there is data on walking and running in the HSE, the location of these activities is not reported so it is not possible to ascertain the frequency of engaging in them in blue space environments. Further, although nationally representative of the English population, this data does not include the rest of the UK.

The second survey, which is representative of the whole of the UK (England, Scotland, Wales and Northern Ireland) is the national Watersports and Leisure Participation Survey (WLPS, Arkenford, 2013). We examine only the latest wave (2013) which included 12,704 individuals. In addition to focusing only on watersports, and including individuals from all parts of the UK, this survey differed from the HSE in that a) it asked respondents whether they engaged in the activity at least once in the last 12 months, as opposed to the last four weeks, and b) it included a broader range of activities that could be classed as blue exercise such as coastal walking. Although frequencies of activities that were also included in the HSE were generally higher, in part due no doubt to the longer time frame and possibly also the inclusion of other UK countries, they were still small in overall percentage terms: sailing (2.3 per cent), rowing/sculling (0.8 per cent), canoeing (3 per cent); surfing (1.3 per cent); wind-surfing (0.3 per cent); scuba-diving (0.6 per cent). Proportions of people reporting other kinds of blue exercise activities were, though, often higher: spending general leisure time at the beach (16.9 per cent); outdoor swimming (10.5 per cent); coastal walking (8.2 per cent); angling (2.1 per cent); cliff-climbing (0.7 per cent); coasteering (0.3 per cent).

Despite the establishment of the Outdoor Swimming Society in 2006, patterns of engagement in outdoor swimming seemed to dip between 2008 and 2012. Specifically, the proportion of people reporting this activity in the last nine years has been between 8–12 per cent, with the lowest numbers in the wettest and coldest summers. The effect of weather is supported by other results in the survey where 88 per cent reported that "better weather" would encourage people to engage in more blue exercise activities. Although still a psychological barrier for some, certain blue exercises in inclement conditions (such as bad weather or cold water) are now less of a factor with the availability of affordable wetsuits.

The WLPS also recognises that not all blue exercise activity recorded takes part in UK waters. Only 49 per cent of participants who reported surfing, for instance, reported surfing in the UK. Further, for some activities, like coasteering, most individuals reported only engaging in it once during a 12-month period, whereas angling had an average yearly rate of 10.6 times (Arkenford, 2013). The WLPS also breaks down the activities by key demographics such as gender, age and socioeconomic status (SES). Generally speaking, engagement in any blue exercise (at least once in the last year) was roughly equal across both genders (male: 29.6 per cent, female: 28.1 per cent), tended to be higher among those aged <55yrs (16–34: 32.4 per cent; 35–54: 32.4 per cent; 55+: 21.1 per cent) and among the more affluent in terms of socioeconomic grouping (AB: 41.5 per cent; C1: 32.9 per cent; C2DE: 21.1 per cent). Of note, some activities were engaged in equally across socioeconomic group, for instance angling: 2.1 per cent by AB, 2.0 per cent by C1 and 2.1 per cent by C2DE. To the extent that angling is good for physical and/or mental health, this suggests that this type of 'universal' activity may help to reduce socioeconomic inequalities in health and wellbeing (or at least not to exacerbate them). By contrast, to the extent that some activities, such as canoeing, are good for health then they may be contributing to growing health inequalities, with the more affluent four times more likely to be engaging in it (AB:5.7 per cent; C2DE: 1.4 per cent).

Limitations in the data, which also apply to the HSE, include a lack of distinction between the diverse blue space environments in which the activities were carried out (e.g. coastal vs. inland waterways). This issue is important because distinct characteristics of different blue spaces may support or inhibit physical activity. These issues can be explored in a third dataset, the Monitor of Engagement with the Natural Environment (MENE, Natural England, 2013). Between 2009 and 2013, some 235,565 people in England were asked in face-to-face survey interviews about leisure visits to any outdoor natural space (including urban parks, countryside and blue spaces, such as rivers and the coast) in the last seven days. Clearly, this much shorter time span is likely to result in lower frequencies than the last month for the HSE or 12 months for the WLSP. Nevertheless, the large sample and data collection across all 12 months means that the spread of activities should be representative of the English population. Since we know of no detailed analysis of this data, the current chapter presents, for the first time, a summary of the relevant findings from the MENE for blue exercise participation.

Of the total sample, 93,770 (39.8 per cent) reported making at least one visit to a natural environment in the previous seven days. For one visit in the last week (randomly selected if multiple were reported) the interviewer asked respondents more detailed questions including the location of the visit (which of the following list of types of place best describes where you spent your time during the visit?). For our purposes the most important locations were three blue landscapes: a) 'A river, lake or canal' (n = 8,137, 8.7 per cent of all visits), b) 'A beach' (n = 6,913, 7.4 per cent) and c) 'Other coastline' (n = 3,616, 3.9 per cent). Respondents were also asked: 'Which of these activities, if any, did you undertake?'; 20 types were offered and respondents selected as many as they liked.

Of the four activities that were directly water-based, fishing was the most popular and accounted for 6.8 per cent of visits to inland waters, 1.4 per cent of visits to beaches and 1.9 per cent of visits to other coast. Watersports accounted for just 2.6 per cent of visits to inland waters, 2.0 per cent of visits to beaches and 2.5 per cent of visits to other coast; swimming accounted for only 0.6 per cent of visits to inland waters, 4.1 per cent of visits to beaches and 1.4 per cent of visits to other coast. The majority of *blue space* visits involved activities by water, rather than in/on/under the water, with walking the most popular. Walking (without a dog) accounted for 46 per cent of visits to inland waters, 41 per cent of visits to beaches and 54 per cent of visits to other coastline. Dog walking in these locations then accounted for a further 28 per cent, 21 per cent and 18 per cent of visits respectively. Other activities reported in the three types of blue space (respectively) included running (3 per cent; 1.7 per cent; 1.6 per cent) and horse-riding (0.2 per cent; 0.3 per cent; 0.2 per cent).

Subsequent analysis looked at the socio-demographic characteristics of those undertaking blue exercise. Fishing was the only blue activity that was engaged in by similar numbers of individuals across the lifespan, with similar numbers of people, as a proportion of the population size, of younger (16–34yrs), middle-aged (35–64yrs) and older adults (65yrs+) reporting angling in the last week. By contrast, compared to those in the 35–64 year age category, older individuals were significantly less likely to engage in watersports, swimming and paddling. Younger individuals (16–34yrs) were more likely to go swimming and paddling. Nevertheless, the oldest age group were most likely to go walking. There were relatively clear socioeconomic (SES) gradients for fishing and watersports. Individuals in lower SES groups were significantly more likely to go fishing and significantly less likely to engage in watersports. There were no SES differences for swimming and very little difference for other beach activities such as paddling. In other words, these activities seem to be open to all, and engaged in by all which might be important for helping to reduce SES-related inequalities in health. It was also clear, however, that the simple activity of walking was significantly less likely among lower SES categories than higher categories in blue space environments.

In summary, despite some inconsistency in the results, the broad patterns of current blue exercise in the UK (especially England) are relatively similar across three major datasets. The main messages are: a) participation in watersports and angling is low in absolute terms; b) on-land blue exercise, e.g. coastal walking, are, however, relatively frequent; c) some blue exercise activities are engaged in relatively equally across genders, ages, and SES groups which may help to mitigate against socioeconomic inequalities in health.

Does living near blue space encourage blue exercise?

One question arises from these analyses: does proximity to blue spaces encourage blue exercise? There is a growing body of evidence, much of it international, to suggest that it does. Bauman et al. (1999) conducted a telephone survey with 16,178 households in New South Wales and found that respondents residing in a coastal postcode were 23 per cent less likely to be sedentary, 27 per cent more likely to report adequate weekly energy expenditure, and 38 per cent more likely to report undertaking vigorous physical activities. The implication is that access to blue space encouraged greater levels of physical activity in general. Several other studies in Australasia report similar findings, especially for walking, although the effects seem stronger for women than men (Humpel et al., 2004a, b, c; Witten et al., 2008). A limitation with this work, however, is that it did not explore where the activity was taking place (e.g. it could be that people who live near the coast just happen to undertake other forms of exercise, e.g. gym-based or tennis) than those inland, rather than blue exercise in particular. Further, it is unclear how these data relate to the UK context where the climate and water temperatures are quite different.

Recent analysis of the MENE has helped in both these respects (White et al., 2014). Examining all respondents between 2009 and 2012 we found that a) individuals who live near the coast are, as in Australia, on average more likely to engage in all forms of physical activity at the coast than those inland, b) residents within 1 km of the coast were 16 times more likely to have visited the coast for leisure purposes in the previous week than those living more than 20 km from the coast, and c) the relationship between proximity and physical activity disappears when we control for coastal visit frequency. In other words, coastal residents appear to be more physically active because they undertake activity on coastal leisure visits, including running along an esplanade for instance, rather than other forms of exercise, such as playing tennis. Intriguingly, however, the positive relationship between coastal proximity and physical activity was only present for regions in the west, but not east of England. Potential reasons could include differences in weather, topography, coastal access or population type.

Taken as a whole, these findings might help to explain the cross-sectional data which suggests that people who live near the English coast tend to report higher self-reported health than those inland (Wheeler et al., 2012) and longitudinal data suggesting that self-reported physical and mental health tend to be higher among individuals in years when they live nearer the coast (White et al., 2013). There is now considerable evidence that physical activity in general is strongly related to both physical and mental health (Bull et al., 2010) so to the extent that living near blue spaces encourages blue exercise, there are large potential gains in public health. An obvious limitation with these epidemiological studies, however, is that they have tended to focus on proximity to the coast, rather than inland bodies of water and waterways which may be easily accessible for more people.

Opportunities for children to engage in blue exercise

Children also engage in, and benefit from, blue exercise. However, although a body of work is emerging to suggest that green exercise may be good for UK children (Reed et al., 2013; Barton et al., 2014; Wood et al., 2014a, b), relatively little work has considered children's blue exercise. Nevertheless, there are some indications to suggest that blue exercise might be important. Although not directly related to exercise, the preference and affiliation literature is important to the extent that preferences may encourage children to interact with water environments which in turn can promote children's health and wellbeing. For instance, similar to research with adults (White et al., 2010), studies have shown that children have a preference for water within natural environments (Zube et al., 1983; Mahidin and Maulan, 2012). Mahidin and Maulan (2012) asked children aged 7–11 years to photograph their preferred scenes in a natural park. The results found that water features, such as streams and ponds, were among the most regularly photographed, suggesting that children may have an affiliation with water. Similarly, Yamashita (2002) found that children in Japan were particularly attracted to images of a water corridor, more so even than adults, possibly suggesting a universal attraction across different cultures.

Further, there is currently concern over health and wellbeing issues such as the high levels of obesity (Currie et al., 2012) and low levels of subjective wellbeing (The Children's Society, 2012) that children are facing in the UK today. Encouraging children to interact with natural environments, and in particular blue space areas, may help to alleviate some of these problems. There are a number of possible mechanisms by which this could occur. First, blue space may be beneficial for children's subjective wellbeing by increasing their mood and reducing stress. Ashbullby et al. (2013) interviewed 15 families, discussing leisure time, including the use of coastal environments, with both parents and children individually. Family beach visits were described as relaxing, calming and stress-relieving, and overall the main reasons for visiting were framed in terms of being beneficial for the psychological and mental health of both parents and children and as a way of building positive intra-family relationships. Children also reported experiencing fun at the beach, with exciting activities, such as playing in rock pools and swimming. Another study, where two researchers observed and monitored children in an aquarium setting, found that the longer children stayed at a large fish exhibit the calmer they appeared to be (Cocker, 2012). They were also rated as having a more positive mood the longer they stayed. This preliminary research seems to suggest that blue space environments may, at least, have a positive impact on children's psychological wellbeing.

Blue space may also provide an environment where children can play or be physically active. Ashbullby et al. (2013) found children valued the beach not only in terms of psychological wellbeing, but also because it gave them opportunities for play and physical activity, for example swimming and making sandcastles. Beaches have also been highlighted as more tactile, sensory spaces for children than those commonly encountered in other day-to-day places, offering opportunities for closer interaction with the natural world (Tunstall and Penning-Rowsell, 1998). This is supported by research exploring the relationships children have with local urban rivers in London (Tapsell et al., 2001; Tunstall et al., 2004). It was found that children expressed enjoyment at being able to play in and around the river (Tapsell et al., 2001), carrying out activities such as paddling, splashing and exploring. Another advantage of this space was that it provided a play-space in the surrounding area as well as in the river itself, for example, children could climb in the trees at the side of the river.

Due to the potential benefits of children spending time in blue space, there is a growing movement to utilise these environments for interventions aimed at particular groups of children. For instance, we have been working with GB Boardriders in Cornwall, to examine the potential health and wellbeing benefits of a surf-related programme of activity for children who have been, or are at high risk of being, excluded from school. Our analysis suggested that engagement in this 12-week programme was not only associated with indices of improved fitness (e.g. a significant drop in average resting heart rate), it also improved self-reported satisfaction with one's body image (especially important in early teenage years) and friendships. Teachers also rated participants more highly in terms of social skills and motivation after the intervention (although not more empathic or self-aware). Although it is unclear whether these outcomes are directly linked to the blue exercise component, as opposed to any type of physical activity outdoors, participants frequently cited being in and around the water as a key part of their enjoyment (and willingness to complete the programme) in qualitative interviews. Further work, including better designed studies that directly compare green and blue exercise for children, are now needed to unpack these issues.

Conclusions

We have considered the recent history surrounding blue exercise in the UK as well as a review of current data. Though relatively few people actually engage in water-based exercise when visiting blue space environments, the absolute number may still have important public health benefits in terms of the associated physical activity. Moreover, blue space environments may act as magnets for on-land exercise, such as walks along rivers or playing on the beach. Our review also highlights that living near blue space is, perhaps unsurprisingly, associated with more blue exercise in general, though there may be important regional differences across the country that require further exploration. Further, the blue exercise literature with respect to children lags behind its green exercise counterpart. In particular we now need carefully designed studies that engage individuals, adults and children, in similar exercise within different outdoor settings to begin to tease apart the specific environmental qualities that might be important not only in immediate outcomes, but also with regards to willingness to continue with exercise in the future.

The implications for policy makers are widespread and varied. For instance, the Marine and Maritime Organisation is currently engaged in the development of several marine spatial plans and needs to understand the benefits blue exercise can have on public health and wellbeing and thus the benefits that could be undermined under certain planning options. Further, with new 2015 changes in EU bathing water standards it remains to be seen how the public will react to the new signs potentially warning people against bathing in waters that do not meet the higher standards and whether this impacts the amount of blue exercise being undertaken. Ideally these new standards will drive improvements in water quality and ultimately maintain, and possibly even enhance, the UK's long tradition of using marine and other waters for health and wellbeing.

The writing of the current chapter was supported by the BlueHealth project which has received funding from the European Union's Horizon 2020 research and innovation programme under grant agreement No 666773.

Chapter 8

Forest bathing in Japan

Qing Li

What is forest bathing?

Humans have long enjoyed forest environments because of the quiet atmosphere, beautiful scenery, mild climate, pleasant aromas, and fresh, clean air. These factors combine to induce beneficial effects on mood states (Li et al., 2012). In Japan, a forest refers to land with a tree canopy cover of more than 30 per cent and area of more than 0.3 hectares. The trees reach a minimum height of 5 m with a width of more than 20 m. The main forests comprise Japanese cypress, cedar, beech, oak, and white birch (Li, 2012). Researchers in Japan have proposed a new concept called forest bathing (Li et al., 2007) and assessed its role in preventing lifestyle-related diseases. Incorporating forest bathing into a healthy lifestyle was first proposed in 1982 by the Forest Agency of Japan (Li et al., 2007).

Forest bathing comprises a short leisurely visit to a forest field, called *Shinrin-yoku* in Japanese, to relax and breathe in the phytoncides derived from trees, such as *α-pinene* and *limonene*. This is similar in effect to natural aromatherapy. The term '*Forest Medicine*' represents a new interdisciplinary science, combining alternative, environmental and preventive medicines, to look at the beneficial effects of forest environments on human health (Li, 2012), including: i) increased human Natural Killer (NK) cellular activity, number of NK cells and the intracellular levels of anti-cancer proteins, suggesting a preventive effect on cancers (Li et al., 2007, 2008a,b, 2010); ii) decreased blood pressure, heart rate, sympathetic nerve activity, and levels of stress hormones, such as urinary adrenaline and noradrenaline, in conjunction with increased parasympathetic nerve activity, suggesting a preventive effect on hypertension (Li et al., 2011; Park et al., 2010; Tsunetsugu et al., 2010; Lee et al., 2014) and decreased risk of psychosocial stress-related diseases (Morita et al., 2007); iii) improved mood (by reducing feelings of anxiety, depression, anger, fatigue and confusion and increasing vigour), suggesting a preventive effect on depression (Li et al., 2007, 2008b, 2010, 2011; Li, 2012); and iv) increased levels of serum adiponectin and dehydroepiandrosterone sulfate, suggesting an anti-ageing effect (Li et al., 2011).

Rates of lifestyle-related diseases such as cardiovascular diseases, cancers, type 2 diabetes, chronic respiratory diseases, cerebrovascular disease and hypertension are increasing worldwide. Some 57 million deaths occur annually, with 36 million (63 per cent) due to chronic non-communicable diseases (WHO, 2010). In Japan, the proportion of workers with anxiety and stress has remained at over 50 per cent since the 1980s, suggesting a major mental ill-health challenge. According to the National Police Agency of Japan, more than 30,000 people have committed suicide annually, with depression playing a major role (Li, 2012). The health management of the workforce, especially in relation to stress-related diseases, has become a major social issue and a growing topic in public health. Urbanization, job-related and social stress may contribute to the increases in lifestyle-related diseases (Angkurawaranon et al., 2013; Li and Kawada, 2014). Because forests occupy 67 per cent of the land in Japan, forest bathing is easily accessible. It has also become a recognized relaxation and/or stress management activity in Japan. Therefore, forest bathing, as a tool to prevent disease and promote health has become a focus of public attention (Li, 2012).

People can enjoy the forest via all five senses: the fragrance of the forest, the dominant green colour of the plants, the murmuring of streams and singing of birds, the eating of forest foods and the touching of trees. Ten tips for effective forest bathing have been proposed (Li, 2012):

1 Make a plan based on your own physical abilities and avoid tiring yourself out.
2 If you have an entire day available, stay in the forest for about 4 hours and walk about 5 km. If you have half a day free, stay in the forest for about 2 hours and walk about 2.5 km.
3 Take a rest whenever you are tired.
4 Drink water/tea whenever you feel thirsty.
5 Find a place you like, then sit for a while and read or enjoy the scenery.
6 If possible, bathe in a hot spring after the forest trip.
7 Select the forest bathing course based on your aims.
8 If you want to boost your immunity (natural killer activity), a three-day/two-night trip is recommended.
9 If you just want to relax and relieve stress, a day trip to a forested park near your home would be recommended.
10 Forest bathing is a preventive measure, so if you come down with an illness, see a doctor.

A number of studies have reported the beneficial effects of forest bathing on human health. The nervous, endocrine and immune systems have long been considered independent entities. However, it is now widely accepted that they affect each other through the psycho-neuro-endocrino-immune network. The nervous system affects the endocrine and immune systems by releasing neurotransmitters through the hypothalamus. The endocrine system affects the nervous and immune systems by secreting hormones. Moreover, the immune system feeds back to the nervous and endocrine systems through cytokines (Figure 8.1). Forest bathing has been shown to produce various effects on human health via these interconnected systems.

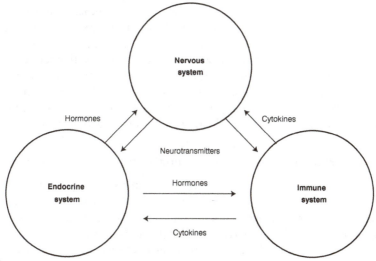

Figure 8.1 The psycho-neuro-endocrino-immune network

Psychological effects of forest bathing

The Profile of Mood States (POMS) questionnaire (McNair et al., 1971) is a 65-item self-administered questionnaire designed to assess six mood states; tension-anxiety, anger-hostility, fatigue, depression, vigour and confusion. We have used this to evaluate the effects of forest bathing in both male and female subjects. Li et al (2007, 2008b) found that a three-day/two-night forest bathing trip significantly improved vigour, anxiety, depression and anger in both males and females. There was no significant change in fatigue or confusion in male subjects (Li et al., 2007); however, fatigue and confusion significantly improved in females, suggesting that women felt more of an effect than men (Li et al., 2008b). A single day trip (Li et al., 2010) and a shorter 2-hour walk (Park et al., 2010; Lee et al., 2011; Li, 2012) in a forest park also significantly decreased anxiety, depression, anger, fatigue and confusion and increased vigour in both male and female subjects. The similarity of these relaxation effects suggests the time spent in a forest setting does not affect the results and a 2-hour walk is sufficient to obtain a positive outcome.

The potential sensory factors influencing mood include olfactory odours such as phytoncides (essential oils) from the trees. Many pine trees emit *α-pinene* (e.g. the smell of Christmas trees). Pinene belongs to a larger family of compounds known as terpenes. These are a huge range of organic compounds, commonly produced by plants. A range of different terpenes are released by various trees in forests. Schiffman et al. (1995) reported that pleasant odours improved the mood of middle-aged males. Both jasmine tea and lavender produced calm and vigorous moods (Kuroda et al., 2005). Aromatherapy-massage with essential oils significantly increased vigour scores (Imura et al., 2006). We previously found that exposure to phytoncides through inhalation had a relaxing effect in male subjects (Li et al., 2009). We detected the phytoncides *α-pinene, β-pinene, isoprene* and *limonene* in forest fields and forest park (Li et al., 2007, 2008a,b, 2010), suggesting that phytoncides from many species of trees may partially contribute to the relaxing effects. In addition, Park et al. (2010) reported that forest viewing significantly increased vigour scores and decreased feelings of anxiety, depression, anger, fatigue and confusion. This was accompanied by a reduction in sympathetic nerve activity and an increase in parasympathetic nerve activity, suggesting that visual factors (the scenery, green colouring) also contribute to the relaxing effects.

Effects on sympathetic and parasympathetic nervous activity

The sympathetic and parasympathetic nervous systems play a pivotal role in the regulation of blood pressure and heart rate: sympathetic nervous activity increases, whereas parasympathetic nervous activity reduces blood pressure and heart rate (Mena-Martin et al., 2006). Heart rate variability (HRV) as well as blood pressure and pulse rate are frequently employed to estimate changes in autonomic nervous activity. The R–R interval obtained from electrocardiograms is used to asses HRV. The power of the low-frequency (LF; 0.04–0.15 Hz) and high-frequency (HF; 0.15–0.4 Hz) components of the obtained heart rate power spectrum for each minute are generally calculated. HF power is considered to reflect parasympathetic nervous activity, and either LF/HF or LF/(LF+HF) is considered to be an index of sympathetic nervous activity (Tsunetsugu et al., 2010). Sympathetic nervous activity also can be determined by measuring the levels of urinary adrenaline and/or noradrenaline (Frankenhaeuser, 1975). It has been reported that forest environments reduce sympathetic nervous activity, increase parasympathetic nervous activity, and regulate the balance of autonomic nerves (Park et al., 2010; Tsunetsugu et al., 2010; Lee et al., 2014). As a result, forest environments reduce blood pressure and heart rate and have relaxing effects (Park et al., 2010; Tsunetsugu et al., 2010; Li et al., 2011; Lee et al., 2014). In addition, these effects indirectly influence the endocrine and immune systems via the neuro-endocrino-immune network, causing a reduction in urinary adrenaline and/or noradrenaline and an enhancement in natural killer (NK) activity in peripheral blood (Li et al., 2007; Li et al., 2008a,b; Li and Kawada, 2011; Li, 2012).

Effects on blood pressure

Sixteen healthy middle-aged male subjects were selected to investigate the effects of forest environments on blood pressure. The subjects took day trips to a forest park in the suburbs of Tokyo and to an urban area of Tokyo as a control in September 2010 (Li et al., 2011). Blood and urine were sampled in the morning, before each trip and after each trip. Blood pressure was measured before, during and after each trip. The day trip to the forest park significantly reduced blood pressure and urinary noradrenaline and dopamine levels, whereas the urban trip did not, suggesting that forest environments, but not urban environments, may reduce blood pressure

(Figure 8.2) (Li et al., 2011). It has been reported that there are significant correlations between blood pressure and urinary adrenaline and noradrenaline levels (Mena-Martín, 2006). We also found that forest environments significantly

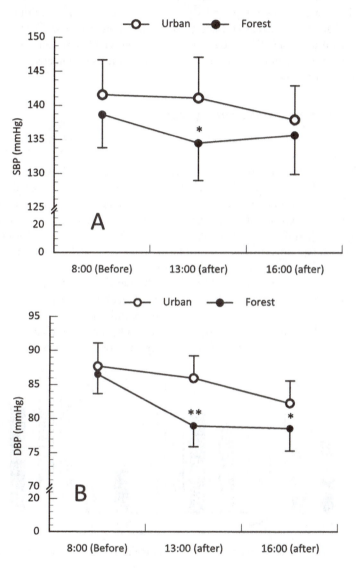

Figure 8.2 Effect of walking in a forest park and walking in an urban area on the levels of systolic (A) and diastolic (B) blood pressure.

Data are presented as the mean+SE (n=16). *: p<0.05, **: p<0.01, significantly different between the forest and urban trips according to the paired t-test. Cited from Li et al. European Journal of Applied Physiology 2011; 111(11):2845–53 with permission from Springer

reduced the level of urinary adrenaline and noradrenaline, suggesting that decreases of urinary adrenaline and noradrenaline contributed to the lower blood pressure. In addition, Mao et al. (2012a) reported that forest bathing had therapeutic effects on hypertension in the elderly and induces inhibition of the renin-angiotensin system and inflammation, thus inspiring its preventive efficacy against cardiovascular disorders. Park et al. (2010) and Lee (2014) also reported that walking in forest environments for about 20 minutes induced small, but significant decreases in both systolic and diastolic blood pressure in young male students compared to walking in urban environments.

Effects on the endocrine system

Forest environments act on the endocrine system to reduce stress hormone levels, such as urinary adrenaline, urinary noradrenaline (Figure 8.3) (Li et al., 2008a,b, 2009, 2010, 2011), salivary cortisol (Park et al., 2010), and blood cortisol (Li et al., 2010; Mao et al., 2012b), inducing a more relaxed state (Li et al., 2007, 2011). Forest environments also significantly increase serum adiponectin and dehydroepiandrosterone sulfate (DHEA-S) levels (Li et al., 2011). Adiponectin is a serum protein hormone specifically produced by adipose tissue; lower than normal blood adiponectin concentrations are associated with several metabolic disorders, including obesity, type 2 diabetes mellitus, cardiovascular disease, and metabolic syndrome (Simpson and Singh, 2008). Levels of DHEA and DHEA-S, the major secretory products of the adrenal gland, decline dramatically with age, concurrent with the onset of degenerative changes and chronic diseases associated with ageing (Bjørnerem et al., 2004; Tsai et al., 2006). Epidemiological evidence in humans suggests that DHEA-S has cardioprotective, anti-obesity, and anti-

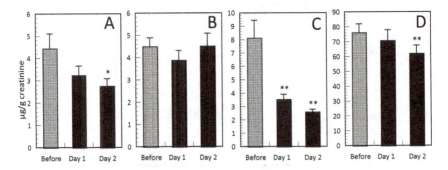

Figure 8.3 Effect of a forest bathing trip on adrenaline and noradrenaline concentrations in urine.

A: urinary adrenaline concentrations in males (n=12), B: urinary noradrenaline concentrations in males (n=11), C: urinary adrenaline concentrations in females (n=13), D: urinary noradrenaline concentrations in females (n=13). Data are presented as the mean+SE. *: p<0.05, **: p<0.01, significantly different from before the trip by paired t-test. Cited from Li et al. Int J Immunopathol Pharmacol. 2008; 21:117-128 and Li et al. Journal of Biological Regulators and Homeostatic Agents. (2008b; 22:45-55 with permission from Biolife).

diabetic properties (Bjørnerem et al., 2004). Mao et al. (2012b) also reported that the concentration of plasma endothelin-1 was much lower in subjects exposed to a forest environment. On the other hand, forest environments did not affect serum estradiol and progesterone levels in females, or serum insulin, free triiodothyronine, and thyroid-stimulating hormone levels in males (Li, 2012).

Effects on the immune system

People with higher NK activity have reported a lower incidence of cancers, whereas those with lower NK activity have reported a higher incidence (Imai et al., 2000), indicating the importance of NK cell function in cancer prevention. In addition, some patients have been shown to have significantly fewer granulysin-positive NK cells than healthy controls; impaired expression of granulysin by NK cells correlates with progression of cancer, and determination of granulysin expression might prove informative for assessing the immunological condition of cancer patients, indicating the importance of granulysin in cancer progression (Kishi et al., 2002). Forest environments have been shown to act directly on the immune system to promote NK activity by increasing the number of NK cells and intracellular levels of anti-cancer proteins, such as perforin, granulysin (GRN), and granzymes (Gr) in both male and female subjects. The increased NK activity has been shown to last for more than 30 days after a trip (Figures 8.4 and 8.5) (Li et al., 2007, 2008a, b, 2010). This suggests that if people take a forest bathing trip once a month, they may be able to maintain a higher level of NK activity. Conversely, taking an urban trip has not been shown to increase NK activity, numbers of NK cells, or the expression of the selected intracellular perforin, GRN, and Gr-A/B, indicating that increased NK activity during a forest bathing trip is not due to the trip itself, but due to the forest environment (Li et al., 2008a). In addition, the percentage of B lymphocytes in a forest bathing

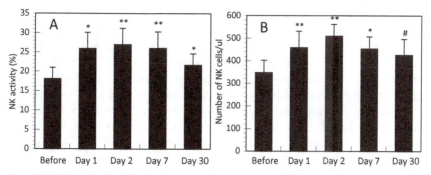

Figure 8.4 Effect of a forest bathing trip on NK activity (A) and the number of NK cells (B) in males. Mean+SE (n=12). *: p<0.05, **: p<0.01, #: p=0.054 different from before the trip by paired t-test. Cited from Li et al. *International Journal of Immunopathology Pharmacology.* (2008a; 21:117-128 with permission from Biolife).

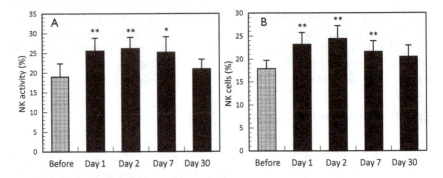

Figure 8.5 Effect of a forest bathing trip on NK activity (A) and the percentage of NK cells (B) in females. Mean+SE (n=13). *: p<0.05, **: p<0.01, different from before the trip by paired t-test. Cited from Li et al. *Journal of Biological Regulators and Homeostatic Agents.* (2008b ;22:45-55 with permission from Biolife).

group has been shown to mildly increase compared with an urban group, which may indicate elevated humoral immunity (Mao et al., 2012a).

Why did the forest bathing increase NK activity? What factors in the forest environment activated NK cells? We have speculated that aromatic volatile substances (phytoncides) derived from trees such as α-pinene, β-pinene, isoprene and limonene play an important role. We detected several phytoncides, such as isoprene, α-pinene, β-pinene, and d-limonene, in the forest parks during the trips. To investigate the effect of phytoncides on NK function, NK-92MI cells, a human NK cell line, were incubated in the presence of phytoncides such as -pinene, 1,8-cineole, d-limonene, and essential oils extracted from trees including Japanese cedar and *Chamaecyparis obtusa*, then NK activity and the intracellular levels of perforin, GrA, and GRN were measured (Li et al., 2006). Phytoncides significantly increased the cytolytic activity of NK-92MI cells in a dose-dependent manner and significantly increased the intracellular levels of perforin, GrA, and GRN in NK-92MI cells. These findings strongly suggest that phytoncides have beneficial effects on human immune function. Thus, we further investigated the effect of tree-derived phytoncide exposure on human immune function in vivo. In the in vivo study, twelve healthy male subjects, age 37–60 years, were selected with informed consent. The subjects stayed at an urban hotel for three nights. Aromatic volatile substances (phytoncides, Li et al., 2006) were produced by vaporizing *Chamaecyparis obtusa* stem oil with a humidifier in the hotel room during the night stay. Phytoncide exposure significantly increased NK activity and the numbers of NK, perforin, GRN, and GrA/B-expressing cells, and significantly decreased the concentrations of urine adrenaline and noradrenaline. These findings indicate that phytoncide exposure and decreased stress hormone levels may partially contribute to increased NK activity. Taken together, phytoncides such as alpha-pinene, beta-pinene, isoprene and limonene from trees may partially contribute to the increased NK activity (Li et al., 2006, 2009).

Furthermore, stress/stress hormones inhibit immune function (Li et al., 2005) and forest environments reduce the levels of stress hormones; therefore, forest environments also indirectly act on the immune system to increase NK activity via the autonomic nervous and endocrine systems mediated by stress hormones (Figure 8.6) (Li, 2010; Li and Kawada, 2011a).

Because NK cells can kill tumor cells by releasing anti-cancer proteins, and forest environments increase NK activity and the amount of anti-cancer proteins, the above findings also suggest that forest bathing has a preventive effect on cancer generation. In fact, people living in areas with lower forest coverage have significantly higher standardized mortality ratios (SMRs) of cancer than people living in areas with higher forest coverage. Additionally, there are significant inverse correlations between the percentage of forest coverage and the SMRs of lung, breast, and uterine cancers in females, and the SMRs of prostate, kidney, and colon cancers in males in all prefectures in Japan, even after the effects of smoking and socioeconomic status

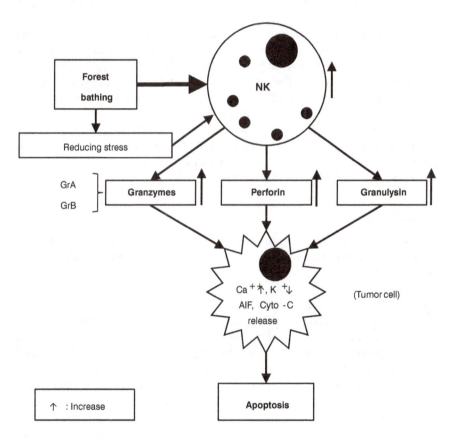

Figure 8.6 Mechanism of forestbathing-induced induction in NK activity

are controlled. These findings indicate that increased forest coverage may partially contribute to a decrease in cancer mortality in Japan (Li et al., 2008c).

Effects on lifestyle-related diseases

Stress may induce and/or exacerbate many lifestyle-related diseases, such as hypertension, ischemic heart disease, gastrointestinal ulcer, and depression (Li and Kawada, 2014). Forest environments can reduce stress hormone levels, such as urinary adrenaline, urinary noradrenaline, salivary cortisol, and blood cortisol levels, suggesting that forest environments may have preventive effects on lifestyle-related diseases mediated by reducing the levels of stress hormones. In addition, Ohtsuka et al. (1998) reported that forest walking can reduce blood glucose levels in diabetic patients. Several reports also found that forest environments reduced the levels of blood pressure (Park et al., 2010; Li et al., 2011; Mao et al., 2012a). Moreover, forest bathing decreases feelings of anxiety, depression, anger, fatigue and confusion and increases vigour, suggesting a preventive effect on depression (Li and Kawada, 2014).

Increasing evidence regarding the beneficial effects of forest bathing on human health has encouraged many research organizations/academic societies to launch projects analyzing the relationship between forest bathing and human health in Japan. The Japanese Forest Therapy Society was established in 2004, followed by the Japanese Society of Forest Medicine in 2007. The purpose of these societies is to promote research on Forest Medicine including the effects of forest bathing and therapeutic effects of forests on human health. In addition, the International Society of Nature and Forest Medicine (INFOM) was established in 2011 to promote research on nature and forest medicine including the effects of forests and natural environments on planetary well-being.

Conclusions

Taken together, forest bathing produces a variety of beneficial effects on human health. The priorities now for governments in affluent countries, including Japan, are as follows:

1   Financially support a large scale longitudinal study to identify the preventive effect of forest bathing on lifestyle-related diseases and cancers.
2   Invest in an international multi-disciplinary research project to compare the preventive effects of forest bathing on lifestyle-related diseases and cancers in different countries (with differing forest landscapes).
3   Assess the therapeutic properties of forest bathing as a preventive intervention to reduce stress-induced diseases.
4   Incorporate forest therapy into the medical insurance system as a new therapy, based on the evidence provided to also reduce medical expenses incurred.

Chapter 9

Healthy parks, healthy people
Evidence from Australia

Mardie Townsend and Claire Henderson-Wilson

Climb the mountains and get their good tidings, Nature's peace will flow into you as sunshine flows into trees. The winds will blow their own freshness into you and the storms their energy, while cares will drop off like autumn leaves. As age comes on, one source of enjoyment after another is closed, but nature's sources never fail.

(John Muir, 1901, p.56)

Introduction

At the recent World Parks Congress in Sydney, Bill Jackson, CEO of Parks Victoria, reflected on changes affecting childhood over the past 50 years. When he was a small boy, he and his siblings were shown the door after breakfast, and told not to come back until dinner time. By contrast, he implied, the young of today are rarely allowed out of their parents' sight and are certainly not encouraged to go bush. Hyperbole or not, the truth is that in Australia (as in most affluent countries) the freedom for children to explore their local wild spaces has all but disappeared. In 2002, Deakin University and Parks Victoria collaborated to publish the first Healthy Parks, Healthy People review of literature (Maller et al., 2002). Drawing on evidence from around the world, this highlighted the importance of parks and nature contact for human health and well-being, not only for children but across the life-span. Second and third editions have followed (Maller et al., 2008; Townsend et al., 2015), making clear that engaging with nature has significant benefits for physical, mental, social and spiritual well-being.

Human relationships with nature

Human relationships with nature can be broadly categorised along a spectrum ranging from ignorance to engagement (Figure 9.1).

At the left end of the spectrum sit ignorance and apathy, resulting in a disconnect from nature and an associated lack of awareness of nature's health and well-being benefits. Typically, at the right end of the spectrum, appreciation of nature is

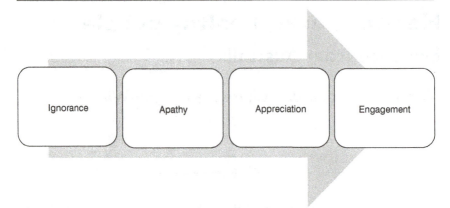

Figure 9.1   Spectrum of humans' relationships with nature

characterised by viewing nature or being in nature (whether actively or passively), whereas engagement with nature is characterised by caring for nature via activities such as pet care, gardening or environmental volunteering. As we move to the right through the spectrum, the level of awareness and connection grows, resulting in greater opportunities for realising the health and well-being benefits.

There are a number of underlying contextual factors affecting the realisation of the health and well-being benefits of nature contact in Australia. Such factors include urbanisation and urban densification, and technological developments.

Australia's population is growing rapidly, with fertility, life expectancy and migration likely to contribute to a doubling of the nation's population by 2075, with a substantial increase in the proportion of the population aged 65 and over (ABS, 2013). Already one of the most highly urbanised societies in the world, much of this population growth is projected to occur in cities. Australia's major cities are already finding themselves forced to adopt measures to contain urban growth and protect green-field sites on the urban fringes (ABS, 2014). This is resulting in urban densification which has flow-on effects in terms of access to parks and nature in inner-city areas (Byrne et al., 2010).

Recently, a report in *The Age* newspaper (Dow, 2014) noted that Melbourne (regularly judged to be among the world's most liveable cities) 'is facing a shortage of public parks and sporting grounds, as skyscraper developers swoop on the city's best blocks and price government out of the market'. The article drew attention to a case where the developers of an apartment project with 1300 units were only required to provide 100 square metres of open space. In September 2014, Melbourne City Council's open space fund was said to be about $11 million – enough to purchase only 550 square metres of land. Taken together, the lack of affordability of land for open space and the lack of requirement for developers to design adequate open space into their developments presents a growing challenge to urban residents' attempts to gain access to the health benefits of nature through parks.

At the same time, we have seen a burgeoning of information and communications technology. While modern technology offers many benefits to society, it has also been associated with the potential for 'cyber-based overload', resulting in increased stress (Misra and Stokols, 2012), less time spent outdoors (Walter, 2013), especially by children (Pratt et al., 2012), and reduced levels of physical activity (Ng and Popkin, 2012). According to Mackay (2007), this rapid technological change, together with rapid social change has contributed to communal anxiety and risk aversion. This, in turn, has contributed to a significant decline in children's independent access across urban environments in Australia (Whitzman et al., 2009) and indeed, to the amount of time children spend outdoors. According to Griffin Longley, CEO of Nature Play WA, 'the average Australian child spends less time outdoors than a maximum security prisoner' (Government of South Australia, 2014).

But it is not only children's use of outdoor spaces which has changed over recent years. The same social changes which have affected children's access to nature, combined with factors such as recent increases in women's workforce participation in Australia (ABS, 2012) and changing perceptions of neighbourhood safety and sense of community, may also be affecting the use of outdoor spaces by adults, particularly women and older people (Francis et al., 2012a).

Not surprisingly, given this context, the physical and mental health of Australians seems to be increasingly under threat. The Australian Institute of Health and Welfare (2013) reported that three in five Australian adults and one in four children are overweight or obese. In terms of mental health, in their most recent report on the prevalence of mental illness in Australia, ABS (2008) reports that 45 per cent of Australians aged 16–85 have experienced a mental disorder at some time in their life, and 20 per cent of Australians experienced a mental disorder in the 12 months prior to the survey.

Australian evidence on 'healthy parks, healthy people'

One of the key determinants of physical health, and especially of levels of overweightness and obesity, is physical activity. A study conducted on behalf of private health insurer Medibank Private in 2008 (KPMG-Econtech, 2008) estimated the total annual economic cost of physical inactivity in Australia at $13.8 billion. Both higher rates of physical activity and lower rates of obesity have been shown to be associated with time spent outdoors (Cleland et al., 2008). So how can we encourage people to spend more time being physically active outdoors?

Both the accessibility and the quality of parks and public open spaces play a key role in fostering physical activity (Villanueva et al., 2013). For example, research in Melbourne by Crawford et al. (2008) found that public open spaces in neighbourhoods of higher socio-economic status (SES) 'were more likely than those in low SES neighbourhoods to possess a number of features that are likely to support children's physical activity'. Similarly, Giles-Corti et al. (2013) found that attractive local environments encourage recreational walking. They suggested that 'access to well-designed green space may partly influence recreational walking by making the experience of walking more pleasant and enjoyable'. Further research is underway using a natural experiment to examine whether improving a park environment contributes to increased park use and increased physical activity, and to identify which specific aspects of the refurbishment contribute to increased use and activity (Veitch et al., 2014).

Parks and public open space are protective not only in terms of physical health, but also of mental health. Research conducted in Adelaide found that people's perceptions of the greenness of their neighbourhood was linked to their mental health outcomes, with those who perceived their neighbourhood as highly green having 1.6 times higher odds of positive mental health (Sugiyama et al., 2008). Subsequent research conducted in Western Australia found that 'from a mental health perspective, the quality of public open spaces within a neighbourhood appears to be more important than the quantity' (Francis et al., 2012b).

More relevant in the context of this book is the research conducted by Astell-Burt et al. (2013) in New South Wales with more than 250,000 participants aged 45 and over. This research explored the association between green space, physical activity and risk of psychological distress. Interestingly, while clear evidence was found of an association between lower risk of psychological distress for participants who are physically active and live in greener surroundings, no mental health benefit associated with green space exposure was evident for those who did not participate in physical activity. While these results suggest that provision of green spaces can be an investment in preventive health, such investment might be best prioritised to the types of green spaces which encourage active engagement (Astell-Burt et al., 2013).

As well as having inherent health promotion potential, parks and public open spaces can be used therapeutically to promote mental health and well-being. Reporting on the outcomes of a six-week intervention including a twelve-day 'bush adventure therapy' programme in Victoria, Australia, involving a small clinical sample, all of whom experienced serious mental health issues, Pryor et al. (2006) noted that 'All participants identified improvements in their capacity to self-manage symptoms of mental ill health and mental disorders'.

But in addition to mental health benefits, this bush adventure therapy programme also demonstrated benefits for social well-being, as all identified improvements in their capacity to socially connect too (Pryor et al., 2006). We know how important social connection is to human health and well-being. As Wilkinson and Marmot (2003) noted: 'Social cohesion – defined as the quality of social relationships and the existence of trust, mutual obligations and respect in communities or in the wider society – helps to protect people and their health'. The holistic nature of this experience, a 12-day wilderness journey as a group, no doubt contributed to this social connectedness, as the following excerpt (Pryor et al., 2006) highlights:

> …the positive social environment was observed to be crucial to the experience for participants. …It offered a safe and secure experience of relational attachment to both fellow participants and staff. Through living together,

experiences became intensive shared experiences – mutual, respectful, at the same time challenging and nurturing. …Nature provided a different world – the wild spaces and changing terrain offered a different physical, emotional and spiritual place from the constructed urban environment participants had come from. …the physical activity, social connection and nature contact assisted in addressing participants' physical, mental, and social needs.

Over recent years in Australia, as urban areas have become more densely populated and house blocks (traditionally large, with each having a private garden) have become smaller, so community gardens have grown in popularity. Just as the bush adventure therapy programme provided multiple health benefits, including social connectedness, so too community gardens have been shown to benefit health in many ways, including by building a sense of community. Research involving the members of an inner Melbourne community garden (Kingsley et al., 2009) found that the garden was described by members as 'a sanctuary where people could come together and escape daily pressures, a source of advice and social support, and a place which gave them a sense of worth and involvement. Members also identified spiritual, fitness and nutritional benefits arising from participation in the community garden'.

The final dimension of health and well-being is spiritual health. Spirituality has already been highlighted above in relation to the bush adventure therapy programme and the community garden. But Brymer et al. (2010) go even further than highlighting the benefits of nature for spiritual health: they claim that nature is the essential mechanism for enhancing holistic human health and well-being:

At the most basic level humanity is reliant on the natural world for resources such as air and water. However, a growing body of research is finding that beyond this fundamental relationship exposure to the non-human natural world can also positively enhance perceptions of physiological, emotional, psychological and spiritual health in ways that cannot be satisfied by alternate means.

Brymer et al. go on to say:

…optimal wellness is reliant on the effective integration of all the wellness dimensions and spiritual wellness is commonly considered to be central to other wellness dimensions. From this perspective, the nature-based experiences that are most likely to augment optimal wellness are those where a person is exposed to nature in such a way that there is an opportunity for actual contact and feelings of connection.

In keeping with these views, we want to focus on the 'engagement' segment of the spectrum outlined above, presenting some Australian case studies as sources of evidence to support the claim of healthy parks, healthy people.

Engaging with nature, enhancing health

This section draws on two projects in which a variety of population groups have intentionally engaged in hands-on interactions with nature in park and other outdoor settings, in several cases as a deliberate strategy to improve their health and well-being, including physical, mental, social and spiritual aspects. The projects which form the focus of this section include: Trust for Nature – community involvement in conservation groups and 'Feel Blue, Touch Green' – environmental volunteering as an intervention to address depression and anxiety.

Volunteering with the Trust for Nature (now The Nature Conservancy)

A team of researchers from Deakin University collaborated with the Trust for Nature (TfN) to explore the health, well-being and social capital benefits gained by community members who are involved in the management of land for conservation through TfN local Committees of Management (Townsend and Moore, 2005).

The study was centred on TfN groups in six rural and urban-fringe communities across Victoria. The specific groups selected for the study were chosen in consultation with TfN to be broadly representative of the TfN groups across the state. A total of 102 people participated in the study (64 males; 38 females) comprising 51 members of a TfN group and 51 controls matched by age, gender and location. All members of the selected groups were invited to participate in the study, and this resulted in participation by 51 TfN volunteers, and control participants who are not involved in conservation groups were recruited through a variety of community settings such as community centres, libraries, Senior Citizens' Clubs, pubs and shopping centres.

The TfN members had resided in, or been associated with, the area for an average of 35.5 years. The average length of membership of the groups was just over seven years, with many members having been involved from the beginning. Forty-seven per cent of the members were retired, 25 per cent were self-employed, generally in farming, 23 per cent were employed, and two were unemployed. The control participants had been residing in the local area for an average of 27 years. Of the controls, 35 per cent were retired, 31 per cent were employed on a full-time basis, 20 per cent were self-employed and the remainder were employed part-time, except for one control participant who was unemployed.

The study involved the use of both quantitative and qualitative methods to collect information from the TfN group members concerning their motivations for joining the group, the social connectedness of members, perceptions of the benefits they gain from membership of the group, including health and well-being benefits, and basic information about their level of health service usage. Similar information (excluding the motivations for joining question) was collected from the controls. The Pearson Chi-Square test was applied to identify significant differences between the responses of the members and those of the control groups. The study also compared the health, well-being and social capital status of members with that of control group members utilising an adaptation of Buckner's Neighbourhood/Community Cohesion Scale (1988).

The results indicate that involvement in the management of land for conservation may contribute to both the health and well-being of members, and to the social capital of the local community. Overall, the members of the TfN groups rated their general health higher, reported visiting the doctor less frequently, felt safer in the local community and perceived an opportunity to utilise the skills that they have acquired in their lifetime more frequently than the control participants. Male members reported the highest level of general health, and the greatest satisfaction with daily activities. In comparison with their control counterparts, members also reported a greater sense of belonging to the local community and a greater willingness to work toward improving their community. Of equal importance is evidence that involvement in voluntary conservation work constitutes a means of building social capital in rural communities which may help reduce some of the negative aspects associated with recent changes in rural communities, such as population decline and loss of services.

The following quotes from TfN members highlight these benefits:

> It sure does influence my health and well-being – the physical and mental work and just the fact that you go out there and relax.

> It helps your health and well-being because you are active.

> It gives you self-satisfaction and it is a relaxing environment – there's no stress.

> By going into the bush it gives me relief from outside pressures. I can go in there and be totally relaxed.

> It's an interest. When you stop work, you have to replace it and this helps to stop things like depression.

> Because I live on my own it's a social outlet and being around any group of positive people – the psychological benefits are great.

> Since I got involved in this …I know more people in this town than I ever did before.

Based on the findings of this study, it is clear that membership of a land management community group offers an enormous range of benefits to members and the community alike. While the direct benefits include an increase in the physical and mental well-being of those involved, there are also many indirect benefits, such as pleasure, enjoyment and a sense of belonging to community. Of equal importance is the fact that involvement in voluntary conservation work constitutes a means of building the social capital in rural communities which, in turn, may reduce some of the negative effects of recent changes in rural life.

Feel Blue, Touch Green

The 'Feel Blue, Touch Green' project was undertaken by a team from Deakin University in collaboration with Barwon Health, Parks Victoria and Surf Coast Shire, and funded by Alcoa World Alumina Australia through the People and Parks Foundation (Townsend and Ebden, 2006). The aim of this study was to explore the specific potential of nature-based activities for promoting health among people suffering from depression, anxiety and related social isolation.

This study involved use of the Anglesea Heath as a setting for engaging participants in supported nature-based activities with ANGAIR (the Anglesea and Airey's Inlet Society for Protection of Flora and Fauna). Anglesea Heath is located in south-western Victoria, approximately 100 km from Melbourne and close to the major regional city of Geelong. It is the richest and most diverse vegetation community in Victoria, with one-quarter of Victoria's plant species found there, including over 80 different types of orchids. It was initially intended that participants would be drawn from the general community and would self-select on the basis that they consider themselves to be experiencing depression, anxiety and/or social isolation. This method of self-selection was adopted because of time constraints and the desire to avoid a lengthy delay in the commencement of the project, due to complex ethics clearance processes. However, not surprisingly (given the target population), recruitment via self-selection proved difficult. Accordingly, an extension of the time frame for the project was granted, and ethics approval was received for referral of potential participants by local medical practitioners and support workers. Each participant committed to undertake at least ten hours of supported hands-on nature-based activities over a period of 5–10 weeks in the Anglesea Heath setting, with the impacts of the experience on the health and well-being of participants being evaluated. The nature-based activities carried out by ANGAIR (and, therefore, available to project participants) include nature walks, weeding, plant propagation, plant identification, planting, wildlife watching and wildlife counting.

The project involved:

- key informant interviews with relevant professionals to identify barriers likely to inhibit participation in the project and to identify mechanisms for overcoming these barriers;
- training in 'mental health first aid' for the ANGAIR members who are engaged in working in the Heath (in a voluntary capacity) with the project participants;
- implementation of a hands-on nature-based activity programme in Anglesea Heath, including a range of activities, times and levels of engagement;
- provision of opportunities for participants to engage in associated social interaction, through barbecue lunches and the like;
- facilitation of involvement through the provision of transport and child care (where required);

- evaluation (including pre- and post-measures, based on a range of validated scales); and
- formal recognition of the contribution of the project participants to the maintenance of Anglesea Heath through the presentation of certificates of acknowledgement.

A combination of formal and informal strategies was used to evaluate the programme. Informal strategies included participant observation by the project's Research Fellow, and informal conversations during the course of project activities. Formal evaluation strategies captured quality of life, health, well-being and participant experiences of being involved in the activities, through surveys and interviews. Surveys included:

- the SF-36 (short-form health survey) which indicates limitations in activities due to mental and physical health problems, as well as general health perceptions;
- the Kessler Psychological Distress Scale (K-10) – a ten-question survey measuring participants' level of emotional distress during the previous month;
- the Activities of Daily Living (ADL) survey – a nine-question survey identifying the amount of independence respondents have in completing usual daily activities;
- the Medical Research Centre (MRC) Dyspnoea Scale – a brief survey identifying respondents' level of breathlessness; and
- an Emotional State Scale (ESS) adapted from the Osgood Semantic Differential Scale to measure emotional parameters relevant to this project.

The SF-36, K-10, ADL and MRC measures were used at the commencement and again at completion of the project to determine general health status and change in health, well-being and quality of life during the time participants were involved in the project. These measures were used to indicate impacts of the project but did not control for outside influences such as the effects of medication, variations in mood and life experiences outside of the project. The ESS was administered at the commencement and completion of each activity to indicate changes in emotional state across 19 parameters, such as bored vs. interested, worried vs. relaxed and happy vs. unhappy. The scale is sensitive to emotional changes experienced during a short time period and indicated the emotional changes experienced due primarily to activity engagement.

At the completion of the programme, unstructured in-depth interviews were undertaken using a phenomenological approach to record and analyse participants' perspectives on being involved in the project and in nature-based activities in particular.

Overall, the SF-36, K-10, ADL and MRC scales did not conclusively demonstrate a change in health for the participants. It is hypothesised that the relatively short duration of involvement in the activities (around six weeks) may have affected the outcomes on these measures and that longer-term engagement in such activities may detect change.

In terms of the ESS, participants experienced positive emotional change across all activities, with the exception of two participants who experienced negative emotional change in relation to one activity (plant propagation being the particular activity for one participant and nature walk for the other).

These positive results in terms of the ESS were borne out in the in-depth interviews, where participants highlighted a range of positive impacts arising from the programme, including developing skills, taking risks and confronting challenges; improving mental health, confidence and sense of self-worth; positive cognitive changes, and stress and anxiety management; managing depression and depressed mood; improving physical health; building social connections; and improving the natural environment.

Quotes from participants included:

I have been able to participate even when I'm not well.

I developed confidence in this supportive environment because [the project partners] offered gentle encouragement and were supportive.

[talking about nature instead of about worries] takes the tension and focus away from myself … and I forget reality … This natural environment grabs you!

You don't get criticised in the bush – self-criticism, negative criticism does not occur in the outdoors.

I have developed an awareness of clean versus polluted waterways, for example by algae. I have become conscious of what clothes washing powder I purchase …Being in the bush has triggered an appreciation for the environment.

The outcomes of this project indicate that there are many potential beneficiaries of projects of this kind: local ecosystems; conservation and land management groups; health service providers; and individual participants (such as people experiencing depression, anxiety and/or social isolation).

Conclusions

Engagement with nature enhances human health and well-being. As the case studies in this chapter demonstrate, significant health and well-being benefits flow when people are actively engaged with the natural environment. Figure 9.2 depicts some of those key benefits.

But, as the 'Healthy Parks, Healthy People' message implies, this is not just a one-way street: the health and well-being of humans and the health of our

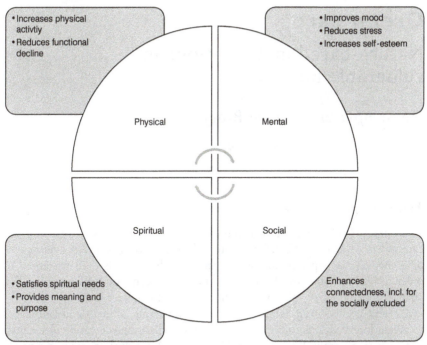

Figure 9.2 Ways in which active engagement with nature (e.g. through environmental volunteering) influences human health and well-being

ecosystems are inherently inter-twined. Aside from all the evidence cited in this chapter (and that is just the tip of the iceberg!), the mere fact of the existence of hundreds of environmental volunteering groups in the state of Victoria, Australia – let alone nationwide and worldwide – suggests that these activities are engaging for humans. And the recent World Parks Congress in Sydney affirmed the benefits of such groups for ecosystem health.

Chapter 10

Green care

Nature-based interventions for vulnerable people

Joe Sempik and Rachel Bragg

Types of green care

This chapter begins by defining green care and outlining the key types of green care available in the UK, before giving a historical overview. An overview of different ways of experiencing and engaging with nature is then presented in order to illustrate the key elements of a range of green care interventions. The chapter concludes by exploring the evidence base for green care.

Green Care has been defined as: '....utilising plants, animals and landscapes to create interventions to improve health and well-being (i.e... not ... a casual encounter with nature)' (Sempik and Bragg, 2013). Recently, though, the newly formed UK Green Care Coalition has refined this definition to 'Green care: nature-based therapy or treatment interventions specifically designed, structured and facilitated for individuals with a defined need' (Green Care Coalition, 2015). The diversity of different interventions is shown under the 'Green Care Umbrella' (Figure 10.1; Bragg and Atkins, 2016).

Social and Therapeutic Horticulture, care farming, and environmental conservation (as a treatment intervention) are the main types of green care currently available, followed by green exercise interventions (such as walking programmes) and Animal Assisted Therapy (including equine-assisted therapy). Other green care interventions exist but are on a smaller scale and so have been grouped together in the 'Other' box. Food growing as a treatment intervention has been grouped with Social and Therapeutic Horticulture as the two approaches share common practices; and Ecotherapy (in its specific sense) has been grouped with environmental conservation as there is much overlap in their practice and ethos (Bragg and Atkins, 2016).

The point made in Figure 10.1 is that each of the interventions can occur in different contexts, with different participants and include a range of activities to suit the needs of those participants. Whilst there is an acknowledged set of practices and pedagogy surrounding these interventions, individual practitioners have the freedom to shape their practice to suit the context and the needs of their clients.

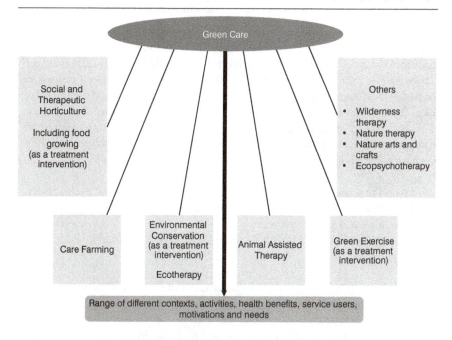

Figure 10.1 The green care umbrella

Source: Bragg and Atkins (2016) adapted from Hine et al. (2008a)

The fundamental elements of green care: an historical perspective

Natural spaces have found themselves alongside places of healing and recuperation. Some of these spaces have been shaped by man into gardens and parks, whilst others have been used as settings to enable the experience of nature – the views, the smells, the sense of 'being there' and sense of place, all contributing to their 'therapeutic' power. A tradition has developed of using the natural environment as a therapeutic setting. The therapeutic quality of nature has been applied to people with many different ailments and difficulties, and gardens (and natural settings) have been used for tending the sick and dying in monasteries, hospitals, asylums, prisons and other institutions.

Walled outdoor areas, known as airing courts, were provided in many hospitals and asylums so that patients could benefit from being outside; shelters were also built in hospital grounds to protect them from inclement weather; and patients were encouraged to work in the farms and gardens not only to help feed themselves but also to breathe the 'fresh air'. Alongside the provision of nature for people with illness and disabilities, there is the long-recognised knowledge that open spaces and nature are pleasing to most people and offer opportunities for many forms of recreation.

The importance of meaningful occupation (as opposed to *employment*) has long been recognised. It is now central to occupational therapy. In writing about the benefits of occupation in the nineteenth century, David Hack Tuke, a descendant of Samuel Tuke, the founder of The York Retreat hospital, advocated occupation as a part of treatment for people with mental ill health, saying that 'the immediate object is not the value of the labour but the benefit to the patient' (Whiteley, 2004, p. 234). In other words, meaningful occupation is more important than productivity. Other reports from that time painted a similar picture regarding occupation but also praised the benefits of fresh air:

> We find that the patients derive more benefit from employment in the garden than anywhere else, and this is natural, because they have the advantage of fresh air as well as occupation
>
> (Nottingham Borough Asylum, 1881, page 11, quoted by Parr, 2007, p. 542).

They also drew attention to the aesthetic qualities of the natural surroundings of the farm, and their ability to stimulate interest and conversation:

> The healthy mental action which we try to evoke in a somewhat artificial manner, by furnishing the walls of the rooms in which the patients live, with artistic decoration, is naturally supplied by the farm. For one patient who will be stirred to rational reflection or conversation by such a thing as a picture, twenty of the ordinary inmates of asylums will be so stirred in connection with the prospects of the crops, the points of a horse, the illness of a cow, the lifting of the potatoes, the growth of the trees, the state of the fences, or the sale of the pigs
>
> (Tuke, 1882, pp. 383-4).

In the mid-1950s, before the advent of antipsychotic medication, O'Reilly and Handforth (1955) noted the importance of social interaction and cohesion in a gardening group for patients with severe mental ill health (schizophrenia):

> Whereas at first each patient went her own way, lost in her own fantasies, there has been a definite trend towards greater cohesion. Verbal and nonverbal forms of communication have increased (p. 764).

Nature appears not only to be pleasing but also a positive influence on well-being and generally desirable. This represents a starting point for much of the research on preference for different landscape types and the psychological effects of experiencing those environments. Whilst much of this work was conducted with people who had no disabilities or difficulties, such research formed the foundations for therapeutic interventions that emerged and evolved from the notions that natural environments and activities within them were 'healthy'. The work of Rachel and Stephen Kaplan

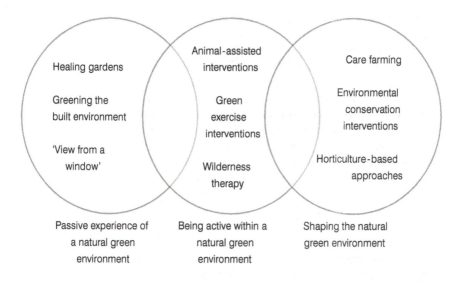

Figure 10.2 Green care approaches and ways of experiencing nature

Adapted from Fieldhouse and Sempik (2014)

(Kaplan and Kaplan, 1989; Kaplan, 1995) on Attention Restoration Theory and that of Roger Ulrich (Ulrich, 1984, 1991) on Psycho-evolutionary Theory (showing that volunteers recovered more speedily from stressful stimuli when they viewed images of nature) were influential in generating momentum for other research – particularly that around effectiveness; and were also instrumental in providing theoretical concepts that were used to explain nature-based approaches as forms of health and social care for vulnerable people.

In order to understand nature-based approaches for health and social care i.e. 'green care', it is useful to consider the different ways in which nature can be experienced. These are summarised in Figure 10.2.

Being in nature

Apart from providing opportunities for passive experiences, the natural environment also offers opportunities for physical activity – 'being active within a natural green environment'. There are many ways in which such physical activity can be taken, for example, through hiking, cycling, boating, climbing and many other pastimes. Whilst these can be recreational activities in which the general public participate, they can also be provided specifically for vulnerable individuals and groups in the form of 'facilitated green exercise'. Research shows that people with mental health problems and learning difficulties are at a much greater risk of physical illness such as cardiovascular disease than the general population (Brown, 1997; Harris and Barraclough, 1998). Outdoor activities can help to reduce such risks through increasing the general level of physical activity and fitness.

The green environment adds to the therapeutic potential of the physical activity. We also know green exercise is effective in promoting psychological well-being (Barton et al., 2012) and is often more effective than exercise alone. Many GPs refer patients to regular exercise programmes in order to help treat conditions such as obesity and diabetes, but whilst some patients engage with these programmes, others drop out. Green exercise programmes offer the additional attraction of their natural settings and may, therefore, increase compliance (Bragg et al., 2013).

Green exercise uses the natural environment as a setting for a range of physical activities. In the course of that process, it inevitably has an influence on the shape of the environment – paths can become established, for example. Such impact is intentionally small and not detrimental – no more than that produced by any other recreational group. It is not the intended aim to shape or change the environment in which the activities take place. However, some green care approaches intentionally shape their environment.

Shaping the green natural environment

The creation of a garden shapes the environment; farming practices shape the environment; conservation interventions shape the environment. These are all examples of green care approaches that are intended to 'shape the natural green environment'. Such interventions use elements of the natural environment, plants and animals, as the fundamental materials for their activities.

The results of such activities, for example, ploughing patterns, garden boundaries, newly established woodlands, can have a profound and long term influence on the landscape and natural environment. It represents a partnership between green care participants and the natural environment. The notion of a partnership is important, it suggests a process of mutual benefit for the individual and the environment. This is the basic principle of *ecotherapy*. Green care interventions have sometimes also been called 'ecotherapy'. However, this is (partly) a misnomer. Ecotherapy is a well-developed set of principles and pedagogy stemming from Roszak's exploration of ecopsychology (Roszak et al., 1995; see also Pedretti-Burls, 2007, 2008). The principle of mutual benefit exists in most (if not all) green care projects but it is not always explicitly stated, and sometimes not recognised. Sustainable practices such as organic gardening, recycling schemes, wind-power and so on are evident in many projects, and participants (both clients and staff) are attracted to them for this reason (Sempik et al., 2005). The important element is that of nurturing – both individual animals and plants, and the whole ecosystem. The opportunity to nurture is a major theme that emerges from the exploration of the therapeutic benefits of green care, for example, as illustrated in the following quote by a participant in a therapeutic horticulture programme: ' We not only nurture the plants, they nurture us as well' (Parkinson et al., 2011, p. 530).

The ways of interacting with nature described here are a general representation, and as can be seen in Figure 10.1, the areas overlap and boundaries become blurred. Some green care interventions straddle those boundaries because those interventions can be modified to suit different individuals with different needs. As seen above, a person can sit quietly in a garden or actively participate in horticulture.

Key elements of green care

One feature that distinguishes green care from casual recreation in the outdoors is its structured nature and defined aims and outcomes. For most people, structure is provided through employment which is the context for meaningful occupation, development of skills and status. Employment provides people with the means (financial and otherwise) of engaging with their community. It enables their social inclusion. Burchardt et al. (2002) have proposed that social inclusion contains four major elements – production, consumption, social interaction and political engagement. These elements are usually provided through employment. Indeed, research over many years has shown that employment provides more than just financial reward; people would still continue to work even if there was no financial need (Morse and Weiss, 1955; Vecchio, 1980). These 'latent benefits of employment' (Jahoda, 1979; Creed and Macintyre, 2001) had been termed vitamins by Warr (1987) and include time structure, opportunities for social interaction, the sense of status that a job and skill provide, common goals and activity. It is well known that loss of employment can lead to severe distress and mental health problems (see Royal College of Psychiatrists, 2008). Such vitamins, therefore, are essential for human health and well-being. However, many of those who participate in green care projects have lost structure and routine from their lives and are marginalised from society due to their illness or disability.

Green care projects give access to those latent benefits of employment for people who are excluded from them and it has been proposed that green care (in the form of social and therapeutic horticulture, care farming and environmental conservation) enables social inclusion (Sempik et al., 2005; Bragg et al., 2013; Bragg, 2014). Indeed, in the study of Sempik et al. (2005), one major theme was 'like employment but without the pressure'.

Historical reports have carefully documented the basic elements that characterise the more interactive forms of green care – meaningful occupation that can include physical activity, an outdoor environment that stimulates interest both in itself and its associated activities, and a social environment that promotes interaction and develops cohesion. These elements, in addition to the notion of mutual benefit discussed above, can be used to create a framework for green care. Furthermore, the mental health and well-being benefits from these 'hands-on' nature-based interventions, stem from the combination of the three key elements; i) the natural environment; ii) the meaningful activities; and iii) the social context, which characterise these green care approaches (Figure 10.3).

These elements of green care can be placed within an Occupational Therapy (OT) model such as the Person-Environment-Occupation-Performance (PEOP) created by Christiansen et al. (2005), and which has been used in the context of green care (Sempik et al., 2010, p. 54).

The model identifies factors relevant to occupational performance and participation and can therefore be used to target areas for therapeutic intervention. The model consists of four elements: the **Person** themselves with their inherent characteristics, strengths and weaknesses; the **Environment** which supplies the factors that support, enable or restrict a person in their activities, tasks and roles; **Occupation** which describes what people want or need to do in their daily living; and **Performance** i.e. the act of doing the occupation. The interaction of these elements determines a person's occupational performance and participation. The environment and the occupation can be adapted to facilitate

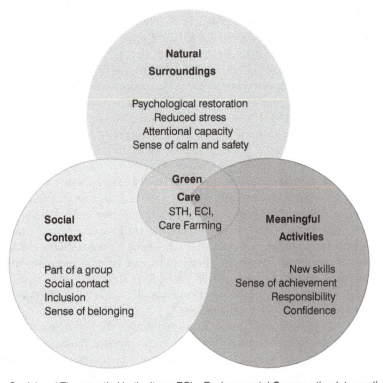

STH – Social and Therapeutic Horticulture; ECI – Environmental Conservation Interventions

Figure 10.3 The interaction of the three key elements within green care

a person's occupational performance and participation. Green care offers many opportunities for occupation (activities) to be tailored to suit a person's needs and abilities, and the natural and social environments provide the context and the stimulus for enhancing occupational performance and promoting participation.

The green care framework has also been mapped to the *Five Ways to Well-being* – a modern initiative developed by the New Economics Foundation and promoted by the National Health Service in the UK (Aked and Thompson, 2011; Bragg et al., 2013). The five ways are:

Connect, Be Active, Take Notice, Keep Learning, Give

Each of these steps could be interpreted through the green care framework shown in Figure 10.3. For example, the process of giving is important throughout green care: the process of mutual benefit to the participant and the environment, central to the principles of ecotherapy, is achieved through giving time and effort to nature, and by avoiding the short cuts and easy fixes of chemical remedies for simple garden problems; social cohesion is formed through the give and take of social interactions.

Developing structured interventions for individuals with a defined need

The previous section has touched upon two frameworks – that associated with employment in general, and that concerned with occupation (as distinct from employment) in a natural environment. These two come together in green care through organised and structured interventions. However, what distinguishes green care from casual recreation in the natural environment, and from nature-based health promotion projects, is not just the organisation and structure of the activities, but the presence of a trained practitioner who facilitates clients' interactions with the natural and social environments and who can set clinical aims and individual goals. The role of the practitioner has often been overlooked when examining the therapeutic effects of green care and instead the focus has been on the natural environment and the associated activities. However, some work has discussed the part that practitioners do play. For example, Elings (2012) has highlighted the relationship between care farmer and client, and compared it to the therapeutic interaction between other treatment providers and their clients.

The role of the therapist or practitioner is illustrated in Figure 10.4. It is important to note that the therapist also interacts with natural and social environments and benefits from such interactions, not only from the 'latent benefits' of their employment but also from participating in green care. They are engaged in the same tasks as the clients and in the same settings, and in some circumstances, for example, in the case of care farming which often takes place in a productive farm, they are working towards the same goals – i.e. running an agricultural enterprise.

It is not uncommon for clients in green care projects to progress to be helpers as their conditions improve, and some may train to become therapists. Often it

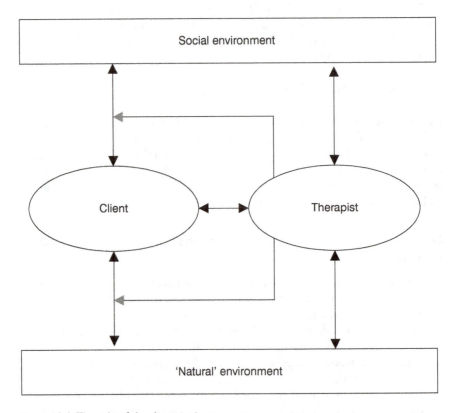

Figure 10.4 The role of the therapist in green care

is difficult to distinguish between clients and helpers (Sempik et al., 2005, pp. 39–43) adding to the general ethos of social inclusion, where the therapists and clients form part of the social environment in green care. Green care projects are often integrated within their local communities and interact with them through, for example, sales of produce or provision of facilities for visitors such as cafés.

Using nature within green care interventions

The preceding sections have laid out the basic structure of green care. It can be seen that it has the potential to improve mental well-being and to enable physical activity in those whose illness, disability, lifestyle or financial means may preclude them from other forms of exercise and recreation. Through the opportunities for meaningful occupation and development of transferrable skills, it addresses the overall functioning of individuals and helps them to interact with the social and natural environments not only of the green care project, but with those in the wider community. Hence, its wide range of indications – green care can improve the lives of people with many different conditions and disabilities. Indeed, it has been used for most if not all vulnerable groups and individuals. By promoting general physical and mental well-being, and creating order and structure for people who may have chaotic lives, it has the potential to reduce the symptoms of conditions such as depression. For example, therapeutic horticulture and care farming have been shown to reduce depression scores in patients with clinical depression (Gonzalez et al., 2009, 2010; Kam and Sui, 2010; Pederson et al., 2011).

Using the frameworks and components above, it is possible to create green care interventions in many different settings (see also: Sempik and Bragg, 2013; Bragg, 2014) and to adapt activities to suit all vulnerable people. The development of interventions has also been subjected to local influences, contexts and resources. Their application and use has also been influenced by local effects. Sometimes the nature of those influences is clear. For example, the use of wilderness in therapy has been developed in the US where there is access to such areas, but is not widely available in Europe.

At other times the local drivers of a particular intervention may not be so obvious. Care farming developed mostly in mainland Europe, it only later became established in the UK even though the UK already had a history of farms and market gardens within its hospitals and asylums. Horticultural therapy was developed in the US in the 1950s and 1960s and quickly spread to the UK in the 1970s but was slower to be used in Europe. Such differential adoption and use of green care interventions may have helped to identify some specific indications for particular approaches. Certain practices have found favour with specific groups or have been found to be useful with people who have particular conditions.

For example, wilderness therapy has been found to be effective for adolescents who have behavioural problems (Wilson and Lipsey, 2000; Williams, 2000). Being in the wilderness gives troubled young people the opportunity to be away from their home environment and to confront personal challenges; it gives them time for reflection. In the UK, both wilderness therapy and care farming have been found to play a similar role for such young people (Hine et al., 2008a; Peacock et al., 2008; Bragg et al., 2013). This does not mean the wilderness therapy and care farming are only useful for young people with behavioural problems but that it represents a good choice of intervention for this group.

Other approaches, such as social and therapeutic horticulture (STH), have been found to have a more generic applicability. This is because they can be used in many different settings, for example, STH can be practised in gardens, allotments and even indoors. It can take place in different contexts such as hospital occupational therapy units, secure units, and projects run by voluntary organisations; and its activities can be adapted to suit a wide range of disabilities. An STH session for people with mental health problems or learning difficulties

Table 10.1 Key client groups of a range of green care interventions

Green care intervention	Key client group											
	Young people	Adults	Older people	Mental health problems	PTSD and stress-related	Drug and alcohol problems	Social difficulties (e.g. long term unemployed)	Behavioural difficulties	Learning disabilities	Physical disabilities	At risk of physical disease (e.g. obesity)	Dementia
Care farming: many different types of farms, and a range of levels of agricultural productivity	✓	✓	✓	✓	✓	✓	✓	✓	✓	✓		✓
Horticulture: includes horticultural therapy; Social and Therapeutic Horticulture; and Garden Therapy	✓	✓	✓	✓	✓		✓	✓	✓	✓		✓
Environmental Conservation interventions: a wide range of settings and activities including:	✓	✓		✓			✓				✓	
'Green Gyms'		✓	✓	✓						✓	✓	
Green Exercise: a wide range of settings and activities	✓	✓	✓	✓		✓	✓				✓	✓
Animal Assisted Interventions: includes Animal-assisted Therapy, Equine-assisted Therapy and Riding Therapy	✓	✓	✓	✓	✓			✓	✓	✓		
Wilderness Therapy: includes Outward Bound programmes and adventure-based learning	✓	✓		✓	✓	✓		✓				

can last for most of the day and take place outdoors, but a session for people with dementia may last only an hour or less and take place indoors, in a residential home or even a secure unit.

Table 10.1 summarises the key client groups of a range of green care interventions. This does not mean the green care is not used with the other groups but the intention is to present an overall picture as to where green care is used in general.

Building the evidence base for green care

The theoretical basis for green care discussed above shows that it may have a range of different effects for different individuals. It is common for mixed client groups, for example, those with mental health problems and those with learning difficulties, to share green care sessions. In terms of practice, this endows green care with great versatility. However, in terms of research it creates some difficulties, especially when such work tries to position itself within a medical literature that sets great store by clearly-defined interventions and homogeneous study populations. Hence, much early work was descriptive or used very small groups. Nonetheless, evidence of effectiveness has continued to emerge since the historical reports and early case studies quoted above. In a 2003 review of social and therapeutic horticulture, Sempik et al. (2003) concluded the following:

> The data presented in this literature review provide evidence for the effectiveness of horticulture and gardening in a number of different therapeutic settings. Experimental evidence from environmental psychology also supports a theoretical framework for therapeutic horticulture. Even though this evidence does exist there is a need for more research and the authors of this review acknowledge the observations of previous writers who have highlighted the scant amount of 'hard evidence' that exists in support of therapeutic horticulture (p.47).

Since 2003, the evidence base has continued to grow and many green care interventions have been researched using a wide variety of research methods. This has enabled some researchers and practitioners to define their 'offer' – what the intervention is, what the indications are, and to list the evidence that supports their claims (see Bragg et al., 2014).

New researchers have also entered the field and brought new methods and approaches. For example, studies have been conducted using randomised (cluster randomisation) approaches (Jarrott and Gigliotti, 2010) and some physiological measures have also been used in this context including measurement of cortisol and heart rate variability (Lee, 2010) and brain imaging (Mizuno-Matsumoto et al., 2008), showing that sophisticated and modern methodology can be applied to research on green care. However, few studies have been conducted using comparative (control) groups, notable exceptions being the work of Christina Gigliotti and Shannon Jarrott on the use of therapeutic horticulture in dementia

(Jarrott and Gigliotti, 2010, 2011); that of Kam and Sui on the use of care farming in schizophrenia (Kam and Sui, 2010); and Pederson's research on the use of care farming in clinical depression (Pederson et al., 2011, 2012a,b).

There are inherent difficulties in studying green care approaches. They are complex interventions which can be difficult to define and standardise between study sites. Even on the same site different individuals may well be allotted, or choose, different tasks and settings; the client population is highly heterogeneous, making it difficult to assemble a homogeneous sample with the same condition or difficulty; and there is generally a slow turnover of clients which has an impact on recruitment of participants (for an exploration of methodology in therapeutic horticulture, see Sempik, 2007). But new research is being conducted and published. Academic study is taking place with doctoral level research on green care in a number of different universities utilising a range of approaches and client groups.

The published research on green care is now sufficiently large and reliable for it to be subjected to systematic review. Annerstedt and Wahrborg (2011) analysed 35 studies and concluded:

> This [systematic] review gives at hand that a rather small but reliable evidence base supports the effectiveness and appropriateness of NAT [nature-assisted therapy] as a relevant resource for public health. Significant improvements were found for varied outcomes in diverse diagnoses, spanning from obesity to schizophrenia. These findings highlight the importance of considering nature as an important resource in mental and public health care and the value of putting further efforts into research of this subject (p. 15).

Whilst the evidence for green care continues to grow, in terms of controlled and randomised trials, the quality of the research does not match that of many medical interventions. In the past, some researchers have argued for a more 'medicalised' approach to nature-based research (see, for example, Frumkin, 2004) with randomised controlled trials (RCTs) and standardised interventions. However, as discussed above, green care is a set of complex interventions that can vary widely between individuals on the same programme. There may be a need to re-evaluate the research paradigm in this area to establish what are the most appropriate (and achievable) methodologies, considering that green care has already become established as a form of social care.

'Standards of Evidence' as proposed by Puttick and Ludlow (2013) may be helpful in this respect and are represented in Figure 10.5. Level 1 is the minimum standard, representing a low threshold and appropriate to interventions in their early stages. As data are collected, there is a progression through the levels, demonstrating causality and external validation. Finally, at level 5, there is demonstrable evidence that the service can be delivered at multiple locations and still produce a strong, positive impact. With regards to green care, we need to decide what approaches and methods we need to take us to the final level of evidence.

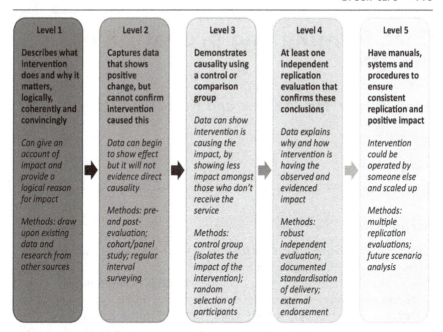

Level 1	Level 2	Level 3	Level 4	Level 5
Describes what intervention does and why it matters, logically, coherently and convincingly	Captures data that shows positive change, but cannot confirm intervention caused this	Demonstrates causality using a control or comparison group	At least one independent replication evaluation that confirms these conclusions	Have manuals, systems and procedures to ensure consistent replication and positive impact
Can give an account of impact and provide a logical reason for impact	*Data can begin to show effect but it will not evidence direct causality*	*Data can show intervention is causing the impact, by showing less impact amongst those who don't receive the service*	*Data explains why and how intervention is having the observed and evidenced impact*	*Intervention could be operated by someone else and scaled up*
Methods: draw upon existing data and research from other sources	*Methods: pre- and post-evaluation; cohort/panel study; regular interval surveying*	*Methods: control group (isolates the impact of the intervention); random selection of participants*	*Methods: robust independent evaluation; documented standardisation of delivery; external endorsement*	*Methods: multiple replication evaluations; future scenario analysis*

Figure 10.5 Standards of Evidence

Source: Bragg and Atkins (2016) adapted from Puttick and Ludlow (2012)

Conclusions

There is a long history of the use of nature as a treatment and as a therapeutic setting for people with a range of illnesses and conditions, and there is much modern research linking the natural environment with positive outcomes in terms of health and well-being. Both this tradition of the use of nature as a therapeutic medium and the findings from that research support the continuing use of green care interventions based around natural settings and the use of elements of nature. Additionally, there has been research into specific green care interventions which has shown that they are effective for a range of individuals with a wide range of difficulties and problems. The evidence base is steadily growing and green care interventions are finding their way into mainstream social care and medical practice. However, the complex character of green care interventions presents many challenges to researchers. Many of the methods and approaches used in conventional medical research, such as randomised controlled trials are difficult to apply in the context of green care. There is a need to take stock of the evidence base, and to establish the best pathways in terms of research and methodology that will lead to the next level of evidence and the wider use of green care.

Chapter 11

Care farming and probation in the UK

Jenni Murray, Helen Elsey and Rochelle Gold

Introduction

Care farms (also termed 'social farms') are utilised by a variety of vulnerable groups in the UK. One such group is adult offenders who have higher levels of poor mental and physical health than the general population (Cattell et al., 2013) and frequently have complex domestic lives. Further, rates of drug and alcohol misuse are particularly high when compared to the general population (Cattell et al., 2013). Interventions that can improve these social and health factors for offenders offer potentially large benefits to the individual and to society as a whole through a reduction in crime rates. Estimated monetary costs of crime vary substantially across countries (Wickramasekera et al., 2015) with UK annual rates ranging from £36–£60 billion.

We outline how probation services are organised in the UK with particular reference to how offenders in the community serve their sentences. This is followed by an exploration of desistence theories (the process of ceasing repeated criminal behaviour) (Manura, 2001) to assess how these inform probation service practice. We then discuss how care farms are applied in community orders, concluding with a section on the theories and evidence relating to care farming and offending. This chapter is informed by our recent research with UK probation services and care farms in England and from a systematic literature review by the authors (Elsey et al., 2014a, 2014b).

Probation services in the UK

Probation services in the UK manage offenders serving their sentences in the community. The service, which has recently undergone major organisational change through a Transforming Rehabilitation Agenda (Ministry of Justice, 2013a), comprises 21 recently formed private Community Rehabilitation Companies (CRCs) and a publicly funded National Probation Service throughout England and Wales. The CRCs are tasked with managing those with a low to medium risk (of causing serious harm) while the NPS manages high-risk offenders. It is envisaged that the new CRCs will encourage innovation with incentivised payment by performance for reductions in re-offending rates. Critical to the success of the CRCs is the use of interventions that have a good evidence base for reducing re-offending rates.

Community orders

The most serious crimes and those committed by serial offenders tend to result in a custodial sentence. Offenders whose crime is considered to be less serious in nature can be given a community order which is completed in the community under the supervision of probation services. A key benefit of community orders is that offenders retain their contact with society gaining benefit from social support but also enabling any re-connections that need to be made with society to be facilitated.

The ultimate purpose of community orders is to reduce the risk of re-offending through 'requirements' – these are interventions that the offender is 'required' to comply with to complete the order successfully. There are many types of requirements (see Figure 11.1) and within these there may be multiple programmes, activities and projects. Offenders can be given one requirement or more depending on the nature of their offence, their offending history, and their lifestyle behaviours. The decision on who receives what requirement is ultimately made in the court but is informed by detailed offender manager assessments with the offenders themselves. Despite the fact that the majority of community orders are managed by CRCs, all community orders are required to include a punitive element. It could be argued that the punitive element presents a tension with the 'rehabilitative' focus implied by the name of the new Community *Rehabilitation* Companies; however, probation services have a duty to protect the public and

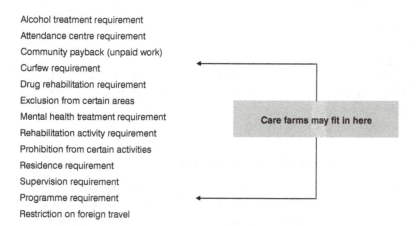

Figure 11.1 Examples of requirements within community orders* and where care farms fit

*Adapted from a number of CRC and Ministry of Justice websites.

must be seen to punish the offender for wrongdoing whilst also having the long-term perspective of reducing re-offending through rehabilitation. The degree to which a community order is punitive is determined by offender needs.

An offender with little or no previous history of offending and no identified needs might be given a predominantly punitive order. An example would include a single requirement 'community payback' in which the offender is required to 'pay back' to the community for harm caused through completion of unpaid work. This can include a variety of projects, such as park maintenance, working in a charity shop, warehouse working and litter picking. Allocation to the various projects is decided by the Community Payback Supervisor alongside the offender. In addition to risk of harm and re-offending, decisions on which unpaid work project an offender is allocated to are also based on, for example, attitude to work, childcare needs, the preferences of both the offender and the project staff, and the gender of the offender. Despite the fact that up to 300 hours of unpaid work may be given to an offender, these types of community orders (where they are not combined with a rehabilitative component) may be regarded as 'light touch', nudging people back into a non-criminal lifestyle (McNeill and Weaver, 2010). Thus although these types of community orders have an overarching punitive flavour they could be looked upon as having a subtle rehabilitative undercurrent as they provide the space to allow people to reflect on current circumstances that might have led them to commit a criminal act.

Community orders that involve an overtly rehabilitative requirement are given to individuals who have particular behaviours that are likely to keep them in a criminogenic lifestyle. These needs may be diverse and include poor education and lack of employment skills, drugs and alcohol misuse, mental ill-health, lack of stable accommodation, poor social support, being part of an anti-social peer group, criminogenic attitudes (beliefs that crime is worthwhile) and anti-social behavioural traits such as impulsivity and poor self-control (Ministry of Justice, 2013b). Commonly probation services provide accredited programmes, treatments (e.g. mental health treatment requirement) or activities in education and training (e.g. activity requirement), alcohol treatment and drug rehabilitation (e.g. alcohol treatment requirement) and in addition offer supervision from an offender manager who can support the offender to find stable accommodation, provide emotional and social support, and help them successfully complete their order.

Factors associated with desistence

Pathways to offending are often complex and individual but in general there are considered to be two main routes: direct, where the person commits the crime to obtain certain rewards; and indirect, where the pursuit of a particular reward incidentally results in criminal activity. Some of the interventions provided in probation clearly target the indirect routes to offending and are known to contribute to desistence – for example through addressing particular needs such as alcohol and drugs misuse (Walters, 1998). However, there are a number of other intrinsic and extrinsic psychosocial factors that are linked with reduced offending behaviour that are more challenging to deliver within individualised interventions. Since repeat offenders can often have multiple interlinked problems, addressing just one factor is unlikely to impact substantially on efforts to desist. Whilst increasing age is also linked with desistance, it is non-modifiable and, therefore, is not discussed in this section. The following are examples of modifiable factors that are closely linked with desistence.

- Having good relationships so that there is a supported social network to which people feel connected or bonded. The bond to society may have been broken through associations with criminal groups and poor lifestyle choices. In younger people this bond with society is most influenced by school, family, peer groups and in older people it is employment, marriage and parenthood.
- For those that want to lead a non-criminal life, having hope and motivation, combined with a belief and confidence that change is possible is linked with desistance (Farrall and Calverley, 2006). Individuals who desist from crime have higher levels of self-efficacy, meaning they see themselves in control of their futures and have a clear sense of purpose and meaning in their lives. These may be concepts that the offender may not have experienced in their lifetime but could be nurtured through mentor support.
- Being able to contribute to and be a part of society is associated with less criminal behaviour.
- Having a non-criminal identity whereby individuals might identify themselves, for example as a worker or a father. This links closely with being part of a social network and contributing to society.
- Being in employment is linked to a sense of mastery and achievement. Again this is closely linked with contributing to society and having a new identity.
- Being believed in so that, for example, others within the network (including probation officers) demonstrate a belief that a non-criminal life is possible.

In addition to these factors it is postulated that a period of reflection and reassessment of what is important to the individual is a common feature of the initial phase of desistance. This period must be accompanied by an opportunity for change as a 'way out' enabling the individual to conceive themselves in a new (and conventional) role (Cusson and Pinsonneault, 1986; Farrall and Bowling, 1999). What is clear from these factors is that the pathway to desistance is a process that can be non-linear. Even if a person re-offends they may still be heading towards a non-criminal lifestyle.

In considering these factors, models have been developed that offer a framework for probation practice.

The first and most established is the Risk Needs Responsivity (RNR) model which targets: 1) factors that predict re-offending to determine who needs a rehabilitative intervention; 2) criminogenic need that determines the nature of the intervention; and 3) cognitive behavioural approaches that aim to maximise the learning, motivation and strengths from the intervention. Critics of this model suggest that the attitudes of offenders towards change and, therefore, their capacity to engage in the responsivity aspect of the RNR model have not been given sufficient attention and, therefore, user engagement is low. A more recent model, the GLM (Good Lives Model) (Ward and Maruna, 2007) aims to support offenders to reconstruct their lives holistically through a positive future-oriented approach that helps them to attain basic human needs, such as autonomy, inner peace and friendships through good choices.

Care farming within a community order

A national survey of care farming in the UK suggested that approximately one-quarter (n=142) of care farms provide support for offenders (Bragg, 2013). As part of a feasibility study exploring the cost effectiveness of care farms for improving quality of life and reducing re-offending in those serving community orders (Elsey et al., 2014b), we contacted a number of care farms to find out about their client groups. What we found suggests that the original number indicated by the previous survey (Bragg, 2013) might be underpinned by a more complex mix of those that used to take in offenders, those that provide support for offenders through, for example, mental health teams (rather than being part of a community order), those that support ex-offenders, and care farms that occasionally work with probation to look after an offender. It is likely that care farms that hold a contract with probation services to take in offenders throughout the year are rare. What is unclear is the extent to which the Transforming Rehabilitation process has had on any contractual arrangements between care farms and probation services. Care farms in the UK that rely on contracts with statutory organisations have, in recent years, been affected by fiscal cutbacks and changes in probation services might equally have led to a rationalising of services to the detriment of care farms.

At the time of writing there were known to be three care farms that had contractual obligations to two CRCs in the UK. A fourth care farm had recently ended its contract with a third CRC. Discussions with care farmers about working with offenders suggest that relationships with probation services can be challenging and this has been exacerbated by the recent organisational changes within the service. Care farmers have also raised concerns that bringing offenders to a care setting where there are other vulnerable groups is not necessarily desirable. One farmer struggled with the concept of providing support to individuals who were ordered, rather than chose, to attend, as is the case with probationers compared to all other client groups. There was genuine concern for how these differences in motivation would affect the organisation at the farm but also the other client groups.

Of the farms that held contracts with CRCs (all of whom were part of our feasibility study), two were provided as community payback and the other two as rehabilitation activities requirements. This arrangement highlights a critical difference in the way that probation services view the role of care farming in the 'rehabilitation' of their offenders. At all farms there was a predominance of men, partly reflecting the fact that crimes are mostly committed by men. National statistics from the Offender Manager Community Cohort Study report a 36 per cent offending rate for males versus 27 per cent for females (Wood et al., 2015). During our feasibility study we found some evidence that at the time of allocation to projects, probation staff steer women to projects other than the care farm because of a perceived male domination at the sites and a need to ensure the safety and comfort of female offenders who may themselves be victims of domestic or sexual abuse. Thus women may not be given a full choice on whether or not they participate in a nature-based activity. However, it is also possible that as offenders are given some choice in deciding their placement, women may be deterred by the perceived physical nature of the work. In studies that have explored the benefits of care farming across a range of client groups there is evidence of a large bias towards males (Elings and Beerens, 2012; Pedersen et al., 2012b; Berget et al., 2008; Iancu et al., 2014).

Care farms as community payback requirements

In the two farms in our study that were offered as community payback, the types of farming activities, the organisation of the farm and the method of supervision were overtly different. One took in offenders that were predominantly low to medium risk of re-offending whilst the other regularly accepted those with a high risk of re-offending.

The first farm, based in the North of England was run as a social enterprise set up specifically to support vulnerable sectors of the population and run on a day-to-day basis primarily by a mental health specialist. The farm had been running for over 10 years with partnerships across local NHS Trusts and the local Probation Service. It was situated on a former landfill site on the outskirts of a large industrialised town with high levels of deprivation. The area as a whole was large but the majority of work took place within a small defined section of the site. A wide range of small-scale activities were offered including working with pigs, chickens and fish, hydroponics, horticulture, manual site maintenance and wood work. The home grown produce was used to prepare a hot meal for the offenders at lunchtime. Although skills gained on the farm were not formally recognised through a skills qualification it was an ambition that the farm was working towards. Supervision at the site was undertaken by on-site staff including a farm manager (the mental health specialist) and an ex-probation member of staff and a reformed ex-offender. Offenders were expected to complete all of their unpaid hours at the farm. Effort was dedicated to establishing manual/professional (such as plumbing or joinery) and social skills sets and physical capabilities of the offenders and planning the group or individual activities around these. The ethos on the farm, as evidenced by their mission statement was one of social inclusion – fitting with society, being valued and equal.

The second farm, based in the South East of England was part of a religious movement. Situated within large grounds that incorporated the Manor House and accommodation, the section that the offenders occupied during their working hours was somewhat segregated. As part of their charitable efforts to feed the homeless, the farm had been set up to provide home grown produce. This farm was unusual in that although it was registered with the Care Farming UK network its primary intentions were not to provide therapeutic activities but rather to obtain free labour as a means to sustain its charitable efforts.

Initially, offenders were sent to the farm on an ad hoc and informal basis but this evolved into a formal and symbiotic arrangement as both the farm volunteer and supervising probation staff observed improvements in offender behaviours whilst at the farm. Unlike the first care farm described above, there was no clear farm manager and although it was a volunteer who organised the days' activities and could be regarded as a farm manager to some extent, it was the probation staff who oversaw the work. Further, the farm would be just one of a number of projects that the offender would be required to attend as part of their unpaid hours so the opportunity to benefit from a close farmer relationship was limited. The range of activities were seasonally dependant but tended to include digging, planting, harvesting, driving the tractor, sweeping the yard and recycling. The only livestock on the farm were cows but because they represent a sacred animal, the offenders were not permitted to work with them. Probation staff would inform the farm staff of any offenders who had existing skill sets that could be utilised by the movement for activities other than those that were farm based. The offenders were offered a hot meal made by the devotees on site at lunchtime. There was no mission statement relating to the therapeutic benefits to its client groups.

Care farms as activity requirements

These two farms worked with the same CRC/NPS area but were geographically quite distant. Based in the Midlands towards the West of England, both farms were long running family businesses. While one had been set up specifically to help vulnerable people, the other had diversified from a traditional farm. Both had mission statements about building social relationships and encouraging change and both provided skills-based qualifications relating to farming activities. Working with livestock was a common activity in both settings with one also offering wood and metal work activities. At one farm there was a post-lunch group reflection session. The provision of hot meals was considered an important part of the day. Transport to the farms was provided by the farmers. This reflects both the rurality of the area and an awareness of the need to support this particularly disengaged group to maximise attendance rates and exposure to the farm environment. At both sites the travel to the farm was considered an important part of building relationships. Both farms celebrated completion of activities through provision of a certificate and a small ceremony. Offenders who were sent there as part of their order, were unemployed, lacked employment skills, and tended to be repeat offenders. Offenders also tended to lack interpersonal skills. The aim was to complete all of the activity in the same setting with the number of sessions ranging from 19 to 22. In general, offenders were also required to attend for supervision sessions at the probation office as part of their community order.

Based on this limited information it is clear that probation services lack a consistent approach to the use of care farms for people on probation. In order to take full advantage of the potential benefits that care farming has to offer this particular group it is clear that probation services need to understand how care farming could contribute to changing offending behaviours and how it fits with desistence theories. This could be facilitated by a two-way dialogue between care farmers and probation to ensure compatibility with each other's individual aims and, therefore, a better fit of the farm within probation service's list of requirements.

Theories of change and evidence of effectiveness of care farming

Although care farming is an overtly practical approach offering multiple activities and opportunities, it is also a complex intervention underpinned by a sophisticated set of theories describing mechanisms of change in social, mental and physical domains. Consideration of the 17 or so theories that have been quoted in connection to care farming (but which are not necessarily specific to care farming) for a range of client groups (see for example Cobb, 1976; Bandura, 1977; Kaplan and Kaplan, 1989; Antonovsky, 1996; Drake and Whitley, 2014) reveals five key concepts (Elsey et al., 2015):

1 The restorative effects of nature – this has particular resonance with the traditional views of mental ill-health but could equally apply to those with chaotic lifestyles that may have troubling thoughts. Through the process of engaging in cognitively non-taxing farming activities the mind is able to relax, reducing the constant bombardment of worries and concerns that interfere with one's capacity to focus on more intensive tasks. Caring for other living things (animals or plants) requires attention but without the burden that comes with caring for other humans. This provides a valuable route to regain the ability to care for and consider others.

2 Being socially connected – Interactions on the farm are not forced, rather they are a by-product of the work on the farm thus they are non-threatening. Lack of trust may be a barrier to offenders connecting socially and the provision of a non-invasive and subtle network of people working on common tasks may ease the pressure associated with environments where social interactions are the sole purpose.

3 Experiencing personal growth – Care farms provide the opportunity to build skills that can impact positively on self-efficacy and with it hopefulness, a concept that is mentioned as a vital precursor to change in the offending literature. As already mentioned, some care farms offer qualifications which

can provide a vital stepping stone to employment. Being in employment is linked with desistence.

4 Being physically active – Over and above the well-known benefits of physical activity for cardiovascular health, farming necessitates physical exertion not as a goal in itself but for the completion of farming tasks. As with social connections, exercise is the subtle by-product of the work. This not only provides an easy distraction for the mind but leads to physical tiredness that is welcome particularly among those recovering from drug addictions and with mental health problems. Gaining a better quality of sleep fosters better coping.

5 Developing a new identity – this links closely to the concept of mental health recovery and relates to changing perceptions of the self and a sense of rebranding through the development of new skills, friendships, and personal growth. Clients may change from seeing themselves as an 'ill person' or an 'offender' to a 'worker' or a 'parent' who can contribute to society in a meaningful way. Opportunities to continue on a voluntary basis on care farms support the continued evolution of this new identity enabling it to become core to who they are.

Amongst these theories there is only one (developed by a care farm team) that suggests explicitly how care farming might lead to changes in offender behaviours. The model suggests that through support to gain vocational and life skills and attain a sense of achievement and fulfilment, offenders can become optimistic and motivated to change leading to a reduction in stress and increase in self-confidence allowing them to make the right choices towards a pro-social life (Evans and Evans, 2015). Although the other existing theories to explain the mechanisms of care farming have not been applied to offenders it is clear that many of the issues that offenders experience are also common to other client groups in particular those with mental health problems and drug and alcohol misuse.

Evidence to support the theoretical mechanisms of change outlined comes from a body of qualitative research on a range of client groups. There have been around 14 studies conducted mostly across Europe that report a variety of findings that appear to provide links between specific activities provided on the farm and perceived changes reported by study participants. How the care farmer uses his skilled judgement of the client's capabilities to set and guide the completion of meaningful tasks features strongly and is linked to clients expressing a sense of being needed, treated normally but with sensitivity to their needs and an increased sense of mastery (Elings and Beerens, 2012; Pedersen et al., 2012a; Kaley, 2015). Likewise working as part of a group enables clients to create strong social bonds built on trust, acceptance, equality and respect (Hassink et al., 2010; Granerud and Eriksson, 2014; Iancu et al., 2014). Being needed, having time away, creating a sense of (new) identity and feelings of belonging are amongst a number of other mechanisms that clients report as positive benefits of being part of the care farming community (Hassink et al., 2010; Granerud and Eriksson, 2014). How these expressed benefits translate to improvements in client outcomes, such as reductions in depression, anxiety, and improvements in quality of life, remain unclear however.

A number of quantitative studies evaluating the health benefits of care farming for various client groups have been reported mostly in the European literature again. A wide range of outcomes have been evaluated within these studies possibly reflecting the different perceived needs of various groups (for example children at risk of exclusion from school versus the elderly with dementia). As a consequence, the volume of evidence for any one group becomes weak. The majority of research studies in this field are uncontrolled before and after studies with high levels of bias such that effectiveness cannot be judged. Only two very small underpowered randomised controlled trials have been reported, one of which contained a highly heterogeneous group of clients with a range of mental health conditions (Berget et al., 2011; Pedersen et al., 2012b). It is not surprising, therefore, that the only published care farm research study involving offenders is a small before and after study. This involved ten prolific offenders (all, therefore, with a high risk of re-offending) and reported that offending rates in the 12 months after attendance at the care farm fell by 65 per cent (Marshall and Wakeham, 2015). The study was challenging to conduct primarily because of the chaotic lifestyles of the offender participants who often did not attend all required sessions. This would indicate that the care farming intervention was powerful enough to need only a limited number of sessions to effect change. Clearly further evidence is required to show that effect is indeed a consequence of the farming intervention but this would require commitment and support from probation services and funding to enable external robust and independent evaluation involving much larger numbers of offenders.

Developing an evidence base for care farming for offenders

Evidence to support the use of care farming for the rehabilitation of offenders is very limited. However, findings from qualitative studies reporting service user experiences do appear to align with the theories that explain the potential mechanisms for change which in turn offer a good fit with the factors associated with desistence. However, more empirical robust evidence is needed in order to test these theories in practice. Due to the limited number of care farm contracts with probation services the numbers required to reliably demonstrate statistically meaningful results would be difficult to achieve. One possibility would be to include other nature-based activity programmes, such as therapeutic horticulture or conservation work, as many of the activities and opportunities that are created on a care farm are similar to these initiatives. So if these kinds of projects were available within other probation services there may still be scope to explore broader nature-based activities for rehabilitating offenders.

Methodologically there are other challenges. The gold standard method for determining effectiveness, the randomised controlled trial, would not be feasible within probation services because of the established and deliberate processes for allocating offenders to requirements. Indeed, even a controlled before and after study would prove challenging in those probation services which offer nature-based projects as a 'rehabilitation activity requirement'. As allocation in this instance is based on a particular need there would not be a true comparator. For example, an offender attending a care farm for social and vocational skills rehabilitation would be unlikely to be comparable to someone attending a drink driving programme requirement. Where the care farm is positioned as one of many community payback (unpaid hours) requirement projects there is more opportunity to identify a comparable group. However, a different challenge exists. Those doing unpaid hours as a punitive order are less likely to have an identified specific need and, therefore, the projects to which they are allocated do not need to deliver on any outcomes other than completion of the order. It is, therefore, unclear what the care farm would be targeting in order to reduce re-offending since rehabilitation is not the aim of the order. Further, since punitive orders such as unpaid hours are considered light touch for those deemed less likely to re-offend the opportunity to impact on re-offending is less.

Despite these challenges there are opportunities. The practice of taking in offenders as part of a partnership agreement with criminal justice organisations is unusual in Europe and in this sense the UK can set an example of innovative approaches to rehabilitation. Indeed, innovation is a key part of the new ethos within the CRCs and as they develop the new companies may be looking to services that can work with offenders on multiple levels in a truly holistic manner – this is where care farming can offer something special over and above many other types of projects. As stated earlier in this chapter, a careful re-examination of the positioning of nature-based interventions within probation would be advantageous, not in terms of matching need with support for the offenders but to encourage a long-term perspective to reduce re-offending and its associated costs. Given that probation services themselves are not research oriented, less robust methodologies (than those required for health service-based interventions) may suffice to ensure the growth of care farming in this sector.

The qualitative evidence that exists conveys very positive experiences offering clear and logical explanations for how being on a care farm brings about change. In this respect, evidence to support the use of care farms for offenders is more advanced than for many other types of community projects. Nonetheless efforts to robustly demonstrate the benefits of care farming for improving key outcomes such as quality of life, mental health and employability still need to be pursued. If conducted outside probation it is likely that the findings of research could be transferable. Connecting up the evidence for care farming between sectors will be an important function to ensure the continued development of the movement to support a wide range of vulnerable groups in society.

Chapter 12

Wilderness and youth at risk

Approaches for positive behaviour change through the outdoors

Jo Roberts, Jo Barton and Carly Wood

Introduction

Much has been written about the value of wilderness and wild places in the healing of vulnerable young people, with some key work occurring in South Africa, Australia, New Zealand and the USA. Writers from Henry David Thoreau, Aldo Leopold and Paul Schneider have long written about the unique qualities that wilderness engenders, such as simplicity and neutrality, enabling humans to re-evaluate, learn, reflect and self-heal. We live in a complex modern world, where young people from all classes and walks of life can find themselves struggling with identity, belonging, and self-management. In affluent countries, as many as one in ten young people suffer from mental ill-health, with young people in lone parent families and families with lower levels of academic achievement being more likely to suffer from mental ill-health (Chief Medical Officer, 2013; Pretty et al., 2015). In addition, youth crime and anti-social behaviour is a continuing problem. In the UK, 12 per cent of all crime is committed by young people aged 10–17 years, with young men being responsible for more than 80 per cent (Ministry of Justice, 2015). An increasing number of young people are also excluded from school. In 2013–2014 nearly 5000 young people were permanently excluded from school and 269,480 for a fixed period; largely as a result of continued disruptive behaviour (Department for Education, 2015).

Wilderness Therapy, *a programme which takes place in a wilderness or remote outdoor environment*, is increasingly used to provide a context for a range of health and development interventions and to tackle youth crime and anti-social behaviour (Wilson and Lipsey, 2000; Connor, 2009). The restorative properties of the wilderness foster personal, social and emotional growth (Davis-Berman and Berman, 1994; Russell, 2001b, 2006a; Norton and Watt, 2014), including significant changes in self-esteem, self-efficacy, confidence, behaviour and decision-making (Cason and Gills, 1993; Hattie et al., 1997; Hans, 2000; Russell, 2006b; Asfeldt and Hvenegaard, 2014; Hoag et al., 2014; Paquette et al., 2014). However, in order for these interventions to have long-term impact, they must lie in sound practice (Russell, 2001). In this chapter we draw on The Wilderness Foundation's *TurnAround* youth at risk programme, which has been running for five years.

The TurnAround Programme

Client group and programme aims

The aim of the TurnAround programme is to engage vulnerable young people to make positive changes in their lives through engagement in nature-based activities. The young people who take part in the programme are typically aged 15–21 years from East England and London and referred from Leaving and After Care Teams, Youth Offending teams, schools and social workers. The majority of the young people have complex needs, are at risk, have had a series of life experiences at a young age which ring out with conflict, poverty of hope and experience, drugs and alcohol abuse, neglect, rejection, lack of safety and love, minimal boundaries, violence and poor aspiration. The programme, therefore, uses the power of nature as a catalyst for change and as a therapeutic place whereby young people can reflect on their life choices and their current destructive pathways (Peacock et al., 2008; Barton et al., 2010; Wood et al., 2012c, 2013b). Throughout the programme young people are engaged in nature-based activities and personal development sessions, such as camping, sailing and open fire cooking in addition to numerous social activities. All these offer a range of skill development opportunities including leadership, planning and organization, social skills, communication and team-work skills. The young people also take part in two wilderness trails which top and tail the experience in locations such as Scotland and Wales. These trails typically last between five and seven days and involve activities such as hiking, wild swimming, and nature watching and canoeing. Participants experience total immersion in nature, whereby they engage in basic living with no facilities, such as electricity or access to mobile phones. The youth are also allocated a mentor whom they regularly meet throughout the programme to discuss employment, education and life after the programme. The overall objectives of the TurnAround programme are to:

i   break down the physical and emotional barriers which inhibit social competence;
ii improve self-esteem, self-confidence, emotional regulation, communication and problem-solving abilities;
iii instil a sense of accountability to the self and others;
iv build trust and team-working skills;
v   educate people to make positive life choices;
vi generate employment and training opportunities and/or further education prospects.

Circle of Courage

The structure of TurnAround is based upon the philosophy and methodology of 'The Circle of Courage' (Brendtro et al., 2005). This Native American Indian rite of passage is modelled on four key elements which are required to ensure individuals have a healthy transition from adolescence to adulthood (Peacock et al., 2007). The model is especially relevant for adolescents experiencing emotional and behavioural problems and has been applied widely in schools, treatment settings and youth development circles. The following four key elements of the circle represent essential growth needs.

i **A sense of belonging**: this is the core value on which the other three elements are based. Humans have a primal need to feel valued and important and belonging to a social group and community plays an influential role in the development of self.

ii **Skills and mastery**: mastering their environment involves developing cognitive, physical, social and spiritual competence, which assists personal growth. Striving to achieve personal goals teaches self-control and responsibility which leads to social recognition and inner satisfaction.

iii **Independence**: refers to developing independence through decision-making, problem-solving, goal-setting, self-discipline and taking personal responsibility for successes and failures.

iv **Generosity**: this factor recognizes the importance of being generous and unselfish, being able to give cherished items to others and making a positive contribution to other people's lives.

A lack of strength in any of these areas is associated with emotional and behavioural difficulties. Thus it is essential that each adolescent progresses through the four phases of the circle to ensure they are a confident and happy adult with a prosocial approach to life. Each element and activity throughout the TurnAround programme, therefore, relates to this circle of courage.

Nature-led consequence and leader characteristics

The understanding that nature-led consequence is a powerful tool also lies at the heart of the work of TurnAround.

One example of this was a wilderness journey on the Isle of Mull, at the start of the winter. Long, dark nights were accompanied by the wildness in nature that winter weather brings. On the first night – groups carrying separate equipment missed each other at a meeting point, and night started to close in. The situation called for an adaptation and coping process as bits of tent were missing, key cooking items were with the other group, and food and drink were unmatched in terms of what would have been a regular meal. To start with, when the situation became apparent to the young people, an initial reaction of anger and tantrums were evoked. Backpacks were kicked down the mountain, swearing, and real frustration and discomfort were evident.

The team leader waited until the initial storming process had played itself out, and then discussed the actions we could take as a group. Stay on the hillside and be cold, wet, hungry and exposed, or, to pull together and take a positive approach and make the best shelter we could and get a brew on for some warmth whilst we look at the next steps of preparing supper. A few hours later, looking at each other over a steaming, rather creative meal, under makeshift cover, we were able to process the experience, learn from the different approaches taken, what worked what didn't, and how to apply this in life back home. It was one of the most effective and powerful reflective group sessions I have ever had with young people.

This example, which included the ultimate natural consequence that you cannot fight darkness and rain, but have to work with it, also included other key elements of our wilderness therapy approach: the facilitation, role modelling and adaptation of the team leader is key to a successful intervention. Responses by the young people in this situation were probably driven by a mix of fear, physical discomfort, and a lack of control. It was deepened by tiredness after a long walk with heavy packs, and potentially unmet expectations. All deeply embedded unconscious and conscious drivers familiar in their everyday life, and for some, typical responses to these, led to the displayed behaviours, anger being the most common.

Through the facilitation of the experience, the leaders, who had been through the same conditions (and in many ways had the same emotions) role modelled coping strategies, resilience, emotional regulation, adaptation and positive actions to resolve a problem. By not responding to the tantrums at play they were able to take on a non-authoritarian approach, which was effective in allowing the emotion to dissipate and to not fuel any further dissent. This approach is characterized as where the leader does not enforce change, but instead allows the environment to influence the individual's response through natural consequences. Staff can step back and let other factors work (Russell, 2001). This kind of emotional intelligence and responsiveness to unexpected experiences is essential to the leader skill set. It is also essential to hold a safe, calm and managed environment as far as possible.

Having had time to get to know the group before the wilderness trail, it is possible to manage more difficult situations because of an existing relationship. This can include situations where some young people hold their leaders in awe as they are the key to their survival. This can cause them to be reactive, rude and combative as a means of holding some control in an environment which has little equilibrium for them, and in the early journey phases they see little benefit from. On the other hand, their relationship with the leaders can be one of compliance and over protection of seeing some of the adult team in ideation. Both have their issues that need careful and sensitive handling.

Excellent safe-guarding training and maturity to maintain a distance that is still close and caring but safe for all concerned is essential for leaders and TurnAround staff, even if seen in simple boundary creation terms. Values that are necessary for the youth to grow, such as resilience, are values that the leaders need to model, whilst not denying their own humanity. This is sometimes a tough position to be in, as often leaders can be taking strain over the five-day journey with little sleep and constant focus on the group. This can, however, be used to an advantage where the generosity factor of Circle of Courage can come to the fore and young people can in turn help adults.

> We had to trek up a steep valley, with a long, sheer drop down into the river gorge to our left. It was hard going through heather and rough terrain and our packs were heavy. I noticed ahead of me, that X had taken his (male) mentor's hand and was helping him up the slope. Discussing this afterwards, this young man who showed little empathy to the world around him generally, shared how he had looked after his mentor when he realized how scared he was of heights, and how good it felt to have been 'in charge' and been in a position to care and help.

Taking these and other factors into account, the adult team needs naturally to relate to the youth in a manner of kindness, loving attention and focus, and to have empathy. This then opens opportunities for young people to respond. This is seen time and time again on trail, that the ethos comes back to the whole group, including the leaders in bucket loads....young people asking caring questions of the adults 'Are you Ok this morning?'. 'Can I help you with getting your pack on?' as examples. The group flourishes when they have fun, are able to laugh and be silly, and there are established processes for group communication around difficult issues, problem-solving, looking out for each other, reflection and decisions.

These kind of behaviours, and the fact that the group is normally in an isolated environment, 'just with each other', helps to make use of a 'family system' approach – with all the norms and values, and expected behaviours of creating a small, tribal group who look after each other, and function effectively to meet basic needs, to be established before and during the journey. Russell (2001) talks of creating a 'nurturing and intense therapeutic process, which helps young people access feelings and emotions suppressed normally by anger, drugs, alcohol and depression'.

> We lie under a canvas roof – sleeping bags touching in the small space that we protect ourselves with from the elusive morning dew, the night, and for them, the unknown.

> In the dark, the conversations start amongst the young people. It is night four or five and our civilised, urban habits are more lost and distant as time has evolved or devolved us. There is a closeness and comfort that has grown over the days. We know much about each other – who sleep talks, who snores, who wriggles...we can read each other's faces, we can feel what they feel.

> 'I would like to live here forever' one says. 'Yes', says another, 'here we are not judged. We have no pressures, it is simple, and peaceful. So different to life back in x. I would really stay here if I could. I think there is no pressure and you can just be yourself. I feel so happy here. You don't really need anything else do you?'.

Silence again as we mull the conversation and it hangs in the air. Slowly we murmur and mumble thoughts and responses and then gradually one by one drift off to sleep or reflection. As a leader – there is a sense of real relief and joy that the wildness is working and is enabling people to evaluate, reflect and consider new ways of being... good messages to try to fall asleep to.

The young people pull close to each other. Sitting in their sleeping bags doing hair, grooming, chatting, sharing, laughing. The guides do their own thing. We watch and enjoy the spectacle and appreciate the easiness so far. We laugh at small things, we enjoy their foibles, funny ways and commentary. We feel tribal again – separate yet together – we have each other – and our group is on its own with no outside impacts.

Behaviour change models

Throughout the TurnAround programme other theoretical frameworks for behaviour change are also incorporated where appropriate, including Neuro Linguistic Programming (NLP) and cognitive behaviour models. Favourite NLP sayings become familiar to the group over the course of the programme – such as 'If you do what you have always done, you will get what you have always done. What can you do differently that would give you a different outcome that serves you better?'.

Work around the cognitive behaviour models of thoughts, feeling and actions, help the group and individuals to understand their own behaviour processes, triggers and responses. They find these models and learnings helpful as often they will express that they don't understand 'what comes over them' when there is an emotional outburst. With the adage of knowledge is power, these tools of understanding their own behaviour drivers empowers change from within, and returns an element of control to the young person where this is often missing. Other approaches used in the programme have been drawn from Transactional Analysis, mindfulness, and Gestalt Therapy but these have been more dependent on the particular training of resident therapists, than endemic to the programme format.

What is, however, embedded in our therapeutic approach is Rogers' (1951) person-centred approach, using reflective language, rapport-building, empathetic responses, and enabling the youth to find their own solutions, as far as possible and is safe in their adventure. This offers satisfaction and ownership of their own outcomes, which is very empowering, builds personal responsibility, and reduces patronage from the adult team to the youth.

Other considerations of theory that are important, include the ecology element of the 'back home' existence of the group in juxtaposition to their current wilderness experience – leaving wide gaps of potential dissonance which the staff work on particularly towards the end of the wilderness journey, and the programme, to address, discuss and seek coping strategies for their group for their return to a world that effectively has stayed the same. They are the ones who have changed and just the knowledge of this can be extremely unsettling and disruptive if not channelled carefully. This element of the facilitation process requires the leadership team to be aware of, and empathetic towards, the often very large differences in their own home lives to those of the young people.

A breakdown of positive behaviour change often occurs at this point in the journey, as the fear and uncertainty of returning home becomes real once again. Where we can often return back to our own homes with a meal and warmth, hopefully family, the young person can often return to a room on their own, no food, no family support and financial hardship.

The end days of the wilderness journeys and the programme as a whole are, therefore, focused on transitioning exercises, reflective conversations and using any tools that help to embed the learning into deeper recesses of the core, where they can be reused and recycled for coping in the future. In addition, preparation of those at home to receive the rather dusty, smelly and changed youth back into their home environment is also provided. Coping tools are offered in terms of the questions asked, how to show interest but not be 'too eager', to allow space for tiredness and some withdrawal.

> From being disruptive, disengaged and highly reactive in our norming and storming first days, X started to relax and draw benefit from the incredible beauty and awe inspiring environment we were trekking through. He was able to work within the team and 'wilderness family', making real contributions in our group discussions that showed his own inner wisdom and strengths. After our five days out we spent two days in a residential setting making sense of all we had experienced and what the young people felt that they had learned and how they could apply these back home. X was emotional about returning home, anxious that he and his mother would return to their normal conflictual relationship patterns and how all would be lost in his mind.

> He wrote his mother an emotional letter of commitment to attempt to start fresh on return and to create a new, potentially good start to their relationship. On return we met his mother in the car park. His face reddened and fell with disappointment as her first words to him were 'You had better have changed, otherwise you are on the street'. There was no welcome home, no interest in his growth, just the repeat of her own defence mechanisms, which lost much of the ground he had covered, and dashed his hopes. For her, nothing had changed, but for him it had been very significant. As staff we could have wept – particularly as we had taken the time to brief all the adults/parents who would be looking after them on return, but also had to understand why and what caused her extreme reaction.

Wilderness journey leaders need to be cognisant of the deeper psychological issues running within their young people and to be adaptive with these processes at play. Not only does the nature-based experience expose more feeling, sensations, emotion, thought, but it can also bring out painful, previously repressed issues. For example, recent work on what is known as Restorative Therapy, shows the inner turbulence of youth who have grown up with a lack of love and trust.

In all behaviour change analysis, which is what we ultimately aim for in all therapy, including wilderness therapy, much of our behaviours are driven from an internal, unconscious process which in turn is linked to our neural pathways and habitual reactions. Changing these pathways, which are generally, fight or flight reactions, is the challenge we deal with. What is interesting is that in this approach, anger, shame, disgust for example are seen as secondary emotions, with the primary emotion being a sense of being unloved or a lack of trustworthiness which links to safety. To break this cycle four steps that can change the unconscious driver and the neural default can be put in place – to say what one feels, to say what you normally do, say the truth, and make a different behavioural choice. All these four elements break patterns and behaviours that are unconsciously led.

Recognizing the powerful impact of these two key drivers, means that if we can ensure that the environment we create on wilderness journeys is as loving as possible, and are determined to be trustworthy as far as we can, then the fight or flight reactivity is reduced. In addition, our focus on group and individual reflection and sharing can help this process and in many instances make use of all four tools for changing neural patterns. Just the juxtaposing of normal life with the wilderness experience opens up different parts of the brain by challenging convention and habit, but mixed with these elements in mind can be even more powerful in supporting change.

Thinking more metaphorically

A regular, transformative and effective tool regularly used within the TurnAround Programme is the use of metaphor, drawing on experiences in wild nature that can reflect a range of life issues. We know that metaphor can be a gentle, depersonalizing mechanism of making sense of deeply personal issues and enables perspectives and understanding that more directive language can fail in. Metaphor also stimulates unconscious processes to come to the fore as they are deemed as non-threatening, and can also be seen to enable different neurological processes to work, drawing on the more creative parts of the brain. For those who spend time outdoors, nature presents myriad opportunities like these and young people can be encouraged to start to think more metaphorically when on wilderness journeys, thus freeing them up and allowing hidden emotion and content to rise to the surface where in safe hands it can be processed and accessed.

> After climbing and abseiling in the bright Pyrenean sun, we made time for solo. Each of us found a quiet place to sit and reflect for around half an hour. The snow glistened off the far side of the valley and the vultures swooped

back and forth over our heads. After some time, X came back down from where she had been sitting and shared with me that a butterfly had flown around her and then come down to sit on her hand. It stayed with her like that for some time. We reflected that she had drawn a butterfly card on our first weekend camp some time ago, which had descriptions of butterflies being a symbol of change and metamorphosis. The significance of her butterfly visit enabled us to talk about her own process of change, what was happening in her own life, and where she felt she was heading. From time to time through the programme she continued to have butterflies fly over her head, settle on her, and be around her – which was really moving for her, and beautiful to see.

Using tension and disequilibrium to facilitate change

Handley (2005) talks about the need for tension and disequilibrium as a means of creating change. Attitudes he writes, 'can only be redirected through an experience of disequilibrium, positive decision making and feedback. New possibilities are created as situations are faced where old perspectives no longer apply. …it facilitates seeing and doing things differently. The TurnAround programme's wilderness experience is the vehicle for this to occur'.

> There is no time pressure today and the group seem resistant to kayak or do much else. There is a need to go with the flow but also to keep focus that we are here to grow and stretch. Fine balance between the two agendas. Part of the experience too is to relax and soften 'life' – to ease the stresses and pressures that so many of these young people live with each day…it is like a metaphor of clay. Too dry and it crumbles as you work with it, soft and moist it is something that can be worked with – to create new forms and to take new shape. We forget sometimes that play is actually learning and growth and something we forget in a structured world.
>
> The morning brings unexpected outcomes. I sit with x and talk – she shares pain and shame spontaneously – there is no pressure for it to be resolved – but in its sharing is a start of its re-evaluation and we are able to work together on seeing some things in a new perspective. As children when things happen to us it is so important to understand that the adults need to take responsibility – not them. Each new wave brings in fresh water on the tide, each new life experience for her, brings new insights.
>
> She almost symbolically throws away elements of her own 'shut down' by choosing to swim in shorts and a strappy top for the first time – perhaps freeing herself of her personal shame and self-deprecation and being liberated and able to enjoy what the world has to offer. And most importantly herself.

Throughout the TurnAround Programme we choose places and ways to work that have disequilibrium naturally within them. The carrying of a heavy pack, the paddling of a canoe or kayak through difficult waters, the needing to dig holes to go to the toilet, the lack of seating other than on the ground, sleeping on thin mats, sometimes the cold, the effort of collecting water, midges, other animals, all add to this process. This is where the magic of the change process lies and the coping mechanisms that take place reduce the normal blockages and habitual behaviours and veneers, and the new mindfulness within the experience can allow the individual to see themselves in a new light. Responsibility lies with each individual in how the programme progresses.

By changing perspectives and attitudes, so do behaviours and actions, and the leaders need to respond and flex quickly to capture the moments, reinforce the learning through praise, feedback and reflections, and to use the group to continue to reward and support these new actions in each other. One of the key pieces of work in TurnAround is to enable the group to do much of the work for itself and its individual young people. In a well-functioning group, there can be far more power in the feedback of youth to youth, than in leader to youth. This evaluation of an individual's progress is critically important. The ability to talk in the group is fostered from the start and is a safety mechanism for individuals and the group itself. Through the group, we establish 'proper ways to manage anger, share emotions, and process interpersonal issues that are modelled in a safe and neutral environment'.

> After we pack up camp and move down to the kayaks for breakfast and tea – we take time for a solo period of about 15 minutes with silence and then feedback. The silence brings comments like 'peaceful', ' relaxed', 'calm' from the group – they get a real sense of this from the exercise which is great.
>
> We then ask them to feed back to each other the strengths they see in each other and what they think others have achieved. We are all moved by what comes out.
>
> Examples like 'she has curbed her anger so well through the week – a major growth point and such a team player', 'x has broken free from her self-consciousness and allowed herself to be free', 'x has been a vital part of the group and shared and engaged with everyone even though his autism is a problem for him', and 'Y has picked himself up when he is negative and moved himself to try things and enjoy them'.

The value of simplicity and connection to nature

Simplicity is another key element to the transformational nature of the wilderness therapy trails used within TurnAround. This relates to what we take, what we need, how we eat, how we sleep and how we live in general. This paring down, the leaving behind of props to hide behind such as mobile phones and watches, creates a very unique time together. Socializing, talking together, cooking, cleaning, preparing kit become the focus for the day, rather than withdrawing behind screens or TV, and losing out on the human interactions we enjoy in the wild. It also reminds us of how little we need to meet our needs and the lack of 'stuff' is liberating and freeing.

Arrival at the base on our first day is hot and stressful. We had little sleep the night before departing – all having to get up at 3am for the airport shuttle.

In the hot, sun filled room in a strange country, with little sleep, we now have to make sense of our new world. We meet our guides and have to work out communal kit, food, essentials, personal things and somehow it all must fit in a bag like a pillow case or smaller.

Most leave behind watches, phones and electronic items into safe keeping for the rest of the journey (as they will get wet), but also most of our clothes go and along with that, our sense of control.

A miracle is when we finally complete packing the kayaks, have distributed kit to hot and tired people, have a practice air kayaking experience on the beach and a safety briefing, and get into kayaks, and our paddles finally bite into the turquoise clear water.

By working in beautiful and awe-inspiring places, having intimate contact with the wild and living simply, participants develop a different relationship with the earth and nature, as well as themselves. We work as a facilitation team to plan the wilderness journeys to be in harmony with nature, rather than to be so raw that nature is a continual enemy, thus helping to find a bonding, archetypal, ancient connection to the land, which in many of us is lost in today's busy, urbanized world. The connection to nature lies deeply embedded in our cellular structure and quickly can come to the fore in the right circumstances. All contact with nature can evoke change, but this takes us back to the primitive within us, a less programmed individual, closer to emotion and feeling, the senses, life force and spirit. The embedded practice of Leave no Trace ethics underpins our commitment to the protection and value of the natural world, but also breeds in the group a sense of respect and responsibility to the outdoors, all of which are transferrable to relationships with humans. We feel this is an important mirroring process of value for life.

Evaluating the TurnAround programme outcomes

Over the last five years, the University of Essex has conducted an independent evaluation of the TurnAround programme outcomes. A mixed methods approach has assessed participant changes in a variety of key parameters such as self-esteem, wellbeing, connection to nature, behavioural strengths and difficulties, hope and hopefulness and mindfulness. The team developed a composite questionnaire incorporating internationally standardized questionnaires alongside qualitative narrative in order to capture the key outcomes of the programme. The questionnaires were distributed at set time points throughout the programme to analyse changes in participants' scores over time. Whilst each yearly programme has often assessed slightly different outcomes, self-esteem has consistently been assessed over the five phases of the programme. Self-esteem exhibits an inverse relationship with depression and anxiety (Orth et al., 2009), is a risk factor for mental ill-health (Xavier and Mandal, 2005; Griffiths et al., 2010) and has been linked with anti-social behaviour and behavioural difficulties (Moksnes et al., 2010). It is also a key aspect of psychological functioning during adolescence (Moksnes et al., 2010) and predicts life satisfaction during adulthood (Boden et al., 2008). Thus, changes in self-esteem during adolescence are of great importance.

Quantitative analysis findings

Evaluation of the impact of the TurnAround programme has consistently shown significant improvements in self-esteem, mood, behaviour, wellbeing, connection to nature and hopefulness (Peacock et al., 2008; Barton et al., 2010; Wood et al., 2012c, 2013b). Furthermore, when data for all five years of the programme are combined, analysis reveals significant improvements in self-esteem from the start to the end of the TurnAround programme (Figure 12.1).

Further analysis of self-esteem also suggests that the initial wilderness trail is of great importance. Not only does the trail result in significant improvements in self-esteem, but participants' self-esteem never returns to its baseline values, despite fluctuations over the course of the programme (Figure 12.2). Thus, the TurnAround programme seems to result in a long-term shift in participants' threshold of self-esteem which has significant consequences for future behavioural choices.

Qualitative analysis findings

In addition to the quantitative data derived from the questionnaires, there is a large body of qualitative data supporting the beneficial outcomes of the TurnAround programme, as demonstrated throughout this chapter. Many positive outcomes on wilderness journeys are those that happen in a moment. We often talk about having to live in the moment, and enjoy brief successes as and when they occur. The fact that some of the key behaviour shifts are quick and flighty does not, however, mean that they are insignificant. Each and every one is the start of a new journey of discovery.

> Without us being able to shout a warning X took a run and dived into the water. She came up sobbing and we realised that she had scraped her stomach on a sharp bit of rock under the surface. Unable to swim back she allowed N (one of our male facilitation team) to help her from the water, to comfort her and ensure she was safe. This allowing a man to be so close to her was one of the most significant moments on her journey. She can now also feel that there are people to rescue her when she is in need and pain, and more importantly that men can look after her without needing anything in return.

There are too many personal examples of this kind of outcome from the experiential nature of the work. The classic outcomes are universally understood – the health and wellbeing from eating good food, exercise, no drugs and alcohol, early up and early to bed patterns, sense of physical and emotional

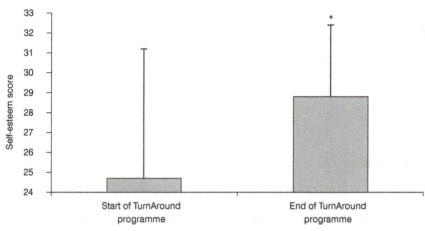

Figure 12.1 Amalgamated changes in self-esteem for the TurnAround Programme (*indicates a significant improvement in self-esteem p<0.01)

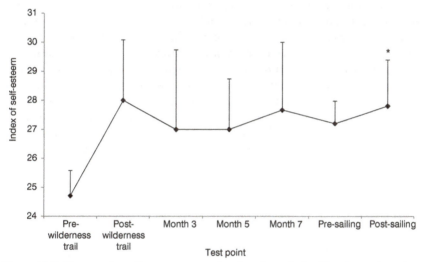

Figure 12.2 Changes in self-esteem over the duration of the TurnAround project (*indicates significantly different from pre-wilderness trail, p<0.05)

accomplishments that are never to be taken away or lost, new skills both socially and individually, evidenced self-esteem growth and personal concept, new attitudes and perspectives, more love to give out and a willingness to receive, positive thinking and a sense of belonging are but some. Other outcomes that need further research relate to the evidence of shifts in neural pathways and the changing of deeper unconscious patterns and beliefs.

A human approach to this work seems to make the difference. Those extra miles driven late at night to get someone home, the consistency of trust and love, the sharing of the experiences together in pain and joy, the soft murmurs as a blood red sun sets and we are all moved by the beauty that lies within our reach if we seek to see it, are the keys to the door for personal progress. Perhaps too it is just the knowledge that you are worth being loved, cared for, and can be trusted and that you can belong in a group, or as part of Gaia, that really matters. For so many people out there who will never have these feelings or experiences, we seek to share widely what we do and to create a respect for wilderness therapy in the health arena so it is more accessible.

Conclusions

The TurnAround programme has successfully enabled vulnerable young people to make positive lifestyle changes through engagement in wilderness trails. Many of these young people were suffering from issues such as low self-esteem and self-confidence, a lack of trust, drug and alcohol abuse and were in need of a strong support network. In addition to promoting improvements in wellbeing, self-esteem, behaviour, nature experience and hope of meeting goals, the TurnAround project also helped participants to make new friends, develop a variety of new skills and develop communication, confidence, social skills and the ability to adapt their behaviour and make positive changes in their lives. Throughout their time on the project participants learnt to communicate with others and developed a sense of achievement from successfully engaging in a variety of activities. The findings of this programme indicate that wilderness programmes may be a successful tool for addressing the growing number of young people at 'risk' of crime and anti-social behaviour and should, therefore, be considered as an alternative option to strategies such as discipline, deterrence, surveillance or imprisonment.

Chapter 13

Green exercise in the workplace

Valerie Gladwell and Daniel Brown

New health challenges are arising in the workplace as occupations become increasingly more sedentary, and workplace stress grows. Both impact directly on health and wellbeing. Workplace interventions that are designed to improve health and wellbeing should provide coping strategies that can directly tackle stress, as well as reducing sedentary behaviours. We explore how exposure to nature can be used as a workplace intervention to reduce stress. We show how green exercise in a workplace setting may be a potentially powerful tool to tackle physical inactivity. We also discuss future research and applications of green exercise in the workplace and identify potential barriers that need to be addressed to increase its future acceptance by both employers and employees.

Increased workplace stress and sedentary time

Much of the waking day is spent within a working environment: approximately 60 per cent of each day over a working life-span of about 40 years (British Heart Foundation, 2009). Although the workplace has been shown to have positive outcomes on physical and mental health (Waddell and Burton, 2006), much work is becoming more mentally demanding, stressful, and also more sedentary due to technological advances within the workplace (e.g. e-mail and world-wide web) allowing employees to conduct most of their work whilst sitting at their desk. Furthermore, non-active transport has become common during the commute to work. The augmentation of stress and sedentary time are negatively impacting on physical and mental health and wellbeing. In Europe, one-quarter of workers say they experience work-related stress for all or most of their working time, with an estimated €136 billion lost to sick leave and loss in productivity across Europe due to mental ill-health (European Agency for Safety and Health at Work, 2014). Increased stress and sedentary time and/or lack of physical activity are workplace challenges that need to be addressed to safeguard not only the health and wellbeing of the employee but also to ensure the maximum productivity (whatever form this may be in) of the company as a whole.

Although, the effect of the indoor work environment on stress has been investigated (Rashid and Zimring, 2008), the formal use of nature and the outdoor environment is almost non-existent. This is despite other evidence to suggest that nature can act as a buffer to stressful life events (Van den Berg et al., 2010). It is well recognised that a work task that is challenging for an employee can cause a rise in arousal/stress levels. This leads to an increase in performance of the task. However, this is only up to a point of optimum arousal/stress before performance begins to decline (Figure 13.1) (Yerkes and Dodson, 1908). The relationship between how much stress/arousal leads to a peak in performance will be dependent on many factors, is individualised and can be task specific. When an employee is unable to cope with the demands of the task that are placed upon them (for whatever reason) their stress levels will be greater and performance affected. Not only does performance decline but at higher levels of stress, physiological changes occur. From an evolutionary point of view, these physiological changes to higher levels of stress were likely to be against a threat of physical danger, such as predators, and were necessary to increase the chances of survival by facilitating a fight or flight reaction. In response to a threat, heart rate, breathing and muscle tension all increase, mainly through the fast-acting sympatho-adrenal medullary (SAM) using the sympathetic autonomic nervous system to release adrenaline and noradrenaline from the adrenal glands. The slower hypothalamus-pituitary-adrenal axis (HPA axis) also plays a part but it is much slower and has longer lasting effects, and these are sustained for a period even after the threat has subsided.

In modern economies, however, the stressor is now predominantly psychological, such as a work task, but a physiological response still occurs. Although, the physiological response may increase arousal (potentially increasing performance as explained earlier), as no physical activity occurs, the physiological responses tend to be disproportionate to what is required. This is particularly relevant if the task

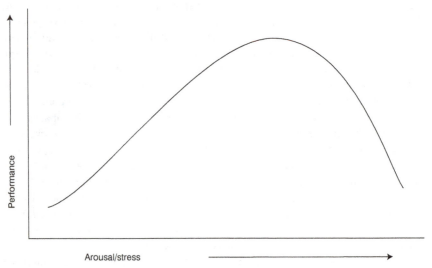

Figure 13.1 The stress-performance curve (adapted from Yerkes and Dodson, 1908)

is considered (or appraised) as a threat rather than a challenge, thus increasing the levels of stress/arousal beyond what is considered optimal for performance. Furthermore, if stressors are repeatedly placed on an employee and there is insufficient time for recovery, the augmented physiological and psychological responses accumulate over time. This more frequent, prolonged and/or severe elicitation of stress responses leads to a detrimental effect on the employee's health by increasing the wear and tear on physiological systems (McEwen and Stellar, 1993; McEwen, 1998). This occurs as with increased levels of stress the body adapts and resets itself, and thus the body operates within a new 'normal' range. This is termed allostasis. A normal response and recovery pattern to stress allows appropriate recovery to pre-stressor levels and the system becomes reset again. However, when there are repeated stressors in quick succession, an inadequate response and/or lack of habituation to a stressor, and/or failure to recover from a stressor, this leads to a continual resetting to new higher levels of 'normal' range. Thus stress, over a period of time, causes chronic exposure to fluctuating or heightened neural or neuroendocrine responses which causes physiological damage to the body (allostatic load) (McEwen and Seeman, 1999).

Stress is amplified with poor social support (from colleagues and management), perceived lack of control, and increased demands. This creates deleterious impact on an employee's psychology and physiology. Stress is, therefore, considered to be an indirect risk factor of ill-health (Kompier and Marcelissen, 1990). However, the negative behavioural and physical coping mechanisms that are utilised by an individual in relation to the stress they are experiencing can influence the direct risk factors of ill-health such as physical inactivity, poor diet and hypertension. An employee who is experiencing stress is more likely to make increased errors in their work, experience a decrease in performance, resulting in an increase in sickness absence. Nevertheless, some employees may continue to be present at work despite illness or mental fatigue (presenteeism) but are likely to display poorer performance. All of these can have an overall negative impact on the whole operation including increases in staff turnover and reductions in productivity.

Positive coping strategies are required to reduce stress levels within a work environment, and to aid recovery and restoration during and between cognitively and mentally fatiguing tasks. These positive coping strategies should lead to a reduction in both psychological and physiological responses to a stressor. Figure 13.2 shows how coping strategies feed into stress appraisal and potentially alter physiological and psychological outcomes.

We know that nature can help provide restorative environments by promoting positive coping strategies, reducing physiology responses, and altering behaviour and cognitive responses. The stress reduction theory (Ulrich, 1981) suggests that as humans have a natural affiliation with nature having been exposed to natural environments for many years, we feel safe in this type of environment. This, therefore, leads to a reduction in arousal, causing relaxation and a decrease in physiological aspects of stress. Therefore, natural environments lower physiological stress. The attention-restoration theory (ART) (Kaplan and

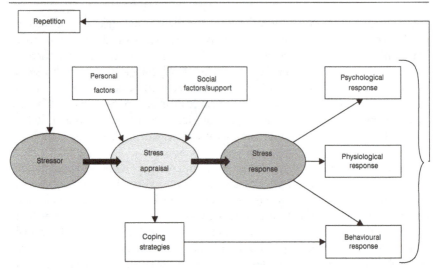

Figure 13.2 Conceptual diagram of the key elements of stress: stressor, stress appraisal and stress response and the influence of personal and social factors and coping strategies

Kaplan, 1989) suggests that humans become mentally fatigued due to increased focus and directed attention. Although, directed attention is vital to undertake work tasks, over prolonged periods of time a person will become cognitively fatigued and unable to maintain their focus. Reduced levels of fatigue can be achieved by changing the focus of an employee's attention from directed attention on the task (which increases levels of fatigue and decreases cognitive function) to more indirect attention. Nature is believed to facilitate indirect attention, creating more effortless brain function, thus reducing directed attention fatigue. Both theories propose that natural environments are restorative and are likely to provide a way to reduce stress, physiological responses and attentional fatigue (which are all applicable to the workplace) and thus help to safeguard health and wellbeing in the long term.

Engagement with nature in the workplace

Research exploring the use of nature in the workplace to improve wellbeing has focused on altering the indoor environment, such as the use of plants within the workplace, views of nature through a window, or the use of images (pictures or screens) showing different natural views.

Integrating nature into the workplace by introducing potted plants can modify mood (Shibata and Suzuki, 2004) and stress levels (Bringslimark et al., 2009) but sometimes the use of plants is not feasible. Views of natural environments from windows have been demonstrated to reduce stress including job stress (Leather et al., 1998), increase job satisfaction and result in fewer reported ailments (Kaplan, 1993). Windows may provide a wealth of opportunities for very brief views of the natural world (Kaplan, 2001). Indeed students who had more natural views out of their windows reported enhanced directed attention during a battery of cognitively demanding tasks (Tennessen and Cimprich, 1995). Interestingly, the type of nature that can be viewed from the window appears to play a role in job satisfaction, with trees resulting in the highest level of satisfaction and mowed areas the least (Kaplan, 2007). However, it appears that no more than a few trees, some landscaping, or some signs of vegetation can all make a difference for restoration. Having buildings present does not seem to impact unfavourably (Kaplan, 1993).

Using images and screens may be a useful alternative as images depicting natural scenes can aid physiological recovery from stress (Brown et al., 2013). Although a surrogate of nature, posters and screens are generally less preferred than real nature (Verderber, 1986), but the use of screens would be of particular benefit in enclosed office spaces without windows or without access to a direct view of nature. This alternative could be considered when technology is already present in the work space or when maintenance of plants is not viable. Furthermore, generally the images presented can be of a higher quality in terms of their nature content than real landscapes from windows and may provide enhanced reduction in stress and restoration.

Modifying the indoor space by introducing images, plants and views only focuses on the immediate employee surroundings. However, encouraging employees to engage with nature on a larger scale can be achieved at set points during the day, such as lunchtime. This brings additional benefits including allowing the employee to be more physically active and spend time away from their work area. However, there has been little rigorous research regarding the benefits of engaging with natural spaces in work time.

Given that nature exposure improves recovery from stress (Ulrich, 1984; Ulrich et al., 1991) and mental fatigue (Berman et al., 2008; Berman et al., 2012); the positive benefits of nature exposure during breaks in the working day is a logical option to explore. However, the use of the outdoors surrounding a workplace has been largely overlooked and yet the green environment has a huge potential for enhancing health and wellbeing. Taking breaks away from the work station to visit natural spaces provides an opportunity to recover from stress and mentally demanding tasks and alter attention to indirect attention. Physically moving from a work environment will enhance the "being away" component of ART, which is particularly important for employees in an office where the work environment is a continuous reminder of the pressure of work commitments.

As only five minutes of interaction with nature has been shown to improve mood and self-esteem (Barton and Pretty, 2010), it suggests the breaks only need to be short to be of some benefit. Furthermore, a short view of nature prior to a stressor in the afternoon, may help improve recovery of the nervous system (Brown et al., 2013). In this study participants viewed a screen with images of nature or built environments for ten minutes prior to undertaking a stressor (which included remembering and reciting numbers whilst being assessed by an investigator). Interestingly, the response to the stressor itself did not change irrespective of the images viewed prior to the stressor. However, the recovery period showed significant differences in the activity of the parasympathetic nervous system, which suggests enhanced recovery of the autonomic nervous system after viewing nature images in comparison to built images. This implies that in a workplace viewing nature at lunchtime might be beneficial to stressful tasks completed in the afternoon. It might also improve recovery between stressors to prevent allostatic load/stress building up over time, facilitating the wellbeing of the employee. More research needs to be conducted to explore this concept further, especially within workplace settings, but it may be that short breaks throughout the day, where the employee is exposed to nature, may be beneficial not only to the employee but the employer may see some gains through enhanced performance and productivity.

An added benefit of taking a break in a natural space for the employee is that they feel they take back some control of the structure of their day. By the employee managing the structure of the day this may help alleviate work-related stress that usually results from the employee not feeling in control. Furthermore, taking the decision to move away from the workplace during a break will, in itself help and be a motivator for being outside and interacting, passively or actively, with nature. In a recent study from Denmark (Lottrup et al., 2012), 37 per cent of workers spent at least one day outside during the working week. The main use of the outdoor environment was to have lunch followed by conversations with colleagues. The majority though, felt that they were not encouraged to go outside (range 77–89 per cent), but with encouragement, mainly by colleagues, increased the likelihood of going outside. Very few (less than 12 per cent) felt that they were encouraged to go outside by their manager.

In a UK-wide survey we conducted in 2011 (n=2079), only 10.5 per cent of workers visited their local green space at work once a week or more, despite 55 per cent rating the quality of local green space around work to be fair or greater than fair. Those that did visit on a regular basis had significantly improved work mood and work engagement. However, there seems to be a gender difference with 6 per cent more men engaging with green spaces than women. It also appears that the relationship between green-space access and stress differs between genders. Reduced workplace stress is associated with increased access for males, but no significant relationship was found for females (Lottrup et al., 2013). Generally the reasons cited for not going outside during a break is that the employee was too busy (Hitchings, 2010), but interestingly seeing others in the space persuaded them to visit more often. This suggests that promoting the outdoors to a few and getting them to encourage others may help foster a culture shift and alter social norms, thus resulting in workplace behaviour change. Therefore, employers should facilitate regular breaks and provide opportunities for finding and using natural spaces, which are accessible in the time frame. Furthermore, by helping a range of individuals (maybe heads of groups) to engage in the outdoors, more employees are likely to take part. Overall, this would be beneficial for the business and would safeguard and potentially increase the health and wellbeing of employees.

The positive outcomes of a break in a natural space are further enhanced as the employee becomes active by leaving their desk; thus breaking up their sedentary time. Furthermore, if breaks within nature involved some form of physical activity such as walking, employees would also be more likely to meet physical activity recommendations, which in turn would lead to further improvements in health and wellbeing.

Physical activity interventions in the workplace

The combination of high levels of stress, longer hours at work, the increasing technological advances whilst at work and the use of inactive transport to commute to work is meaning that there are fewer opportunities to undertake incidental physical activity. Physical activity is a well-known contributor to improved physical and mental health (Bouchard et al., 2006). Some 20 per cent of men and 27 per cent of women aged 18 and over are not meeting World Health Organisation physical activity guidelines of 150 minutes per week of moderate physical activity (WHO, 2010). However, in affluent countries, this figure is elevated further, with 26 per cent of men and 35 per cent of women not undertaking enough physical activity. Furthermore, the higher levels of stress that are reported exacerbate the reduction in physical activity, due to individuals feeling that there is lack of time to undertake physical activity or even take breaks away from their work station (Trost et al., 2002). The periods of time of prolonged inactivity are, therefore, also increasing, which has its own independent negative health outcomes (Hamilton et al., 2008).

All of this together indicates that both pre-emptive and pro-active steps are required to ensure physical activity guidelines are met. The workplace is an ideal setting for this as there is a large target audience. If the cycle of inactivity can be broken and breaks incorporated within a working day then this should reduce stress, diminish prolonged periods of inactivity and increase physical activity. The National Institute of Clinical Excellence recommendations (NICE, 2009) suggest counselling and fitness programmes are the most effective in increasing physical activity levels. This can be achieved through active commutes, active breaks, using the stairs and walking to meetings.

Being physically inactive is a direct risk factor for cardiovascular disease with individuals not engaging in regular physical activity having a 20–30 per cent greater risk for cardiovascular disease (WHO, 2010); thus being physically inactive is a key physical health issue. Walking is a simple activity that promotes sustainable changes in physical activity and helps to reach moderate activity guidelines (Welk et al., 2000). This suggests that walking interventions should be promoted within the workplace (NICE, 2009). Workplace interventions that include walking increase overall physical activity, but it is unclear whether this actually decreases overall sedentary behaviour. Some studies show a decrease in sedentary time whereas others also identified that sitting time is unaffected by workplace physical activity interventions (Chau et al., 2010). However, increasing activity during suitable periods of the day, such as lunchtime, provides opportunities to break up long periods of sedentary time. This may have cardiovascular benefits, even without reducing total time spent being sedentary. This is of particular importance to ensure the health and wellbeing of employees.

A more active workforce reduces absenteeism, reduces health care costs and increases productivity, all of which are likely to aid employers (Proper et al., 2002). Existing research on workplace physical activity interventions have primarily focused on increasing physical activity itself and dietary outcomes, although some have explored other factors. A meta-analysis of physical activity interventions in the workplace showed that participation can have positive effects on fitness and anthropometric measurements as well as work attendance and job stress (Conn et al., 2009). It is important that physical activity interventions in a workplace should not only enhance physical health but also ensure benefits to psychosocial health, to further benefit the employee and the employer. However, only a handful of studies have investigated physical activity interventions and their impact on psychosocial factors (Brown et al., 2011).

The break at lunchtime is a time when employees could engage in moderate physical activity, thus interrupting the long periods of sedentary time. Further, it provides an opportunity to decrease stress levels and restore physical and mental fatigue. However, the lunch break is often a time when employees continue to remain at their work stations due to work demands or peer pressure. Thus a detrimental cycle of increased stress and sedentary behaviour dominates. Physical activity in a natural environment (green exercise) at lunchtime may be of particular benefit for workplace health and could help improve physical and also psychosocial health.

Green exercise interventions in the workplace

NICE guidelines suggest encouraging active breaks to increase physical activity but this guideline should be extended to include active walking breaks within a natural environment. Whilst generic physical activity interventions have been investigated, the use of green exercise interventions at work has received very limited attention. The combination of positive nature breaks and physical activity may offer the opportunity to utilise the physical benefits of exercise combined with the restorative and stress reducing effects of nature, and potentially increase social interactions, thus enhancing psychosocial aspects.

However, only 15 per cent of participants reported using the outdoor environment for physical activity (Lottrup et al., 2012). The quality and accessibility of local green space is important but it may be that individuals require more facilitation to undertake green exercise. The use of green exercise as an intervention in a workplace should require little investment beyond the provision of a walking route and the encouragement for individuals to use it. From anecdotal experience this can be achieved through the development of walking groups that spontaneously arrange and carry out walks during the working day. Alternatively *walk champions* from inside the company can be initiators of walks.

A study that we conducted entitled *Walks4work* (Brown et al., 2012; 2014) demonstrated that a workplace intervention of walking in nature (which included parkland, trees and more natural areas) improved mental wellbeing, reduced negative mood and reduced perceived stress levels in contrast to walking in a built environment (composed of paved footpaths adjacent to roads, housing estates, and industrial areas). The *Walks4work* intervention consisted of an eight-week phase where participants (33 per group) were assigned to one of the two walking groups and were asked to complete two lunchtime walks every week. Both walking groups followed a set circular walking route approximately 2 km in length, designed to provide a walk of approximately 20 minutes in duration. Each participant was free to choose which two weekdays they walked in order to promote adherence and were able to walk individually or with others in either direction around the prescribed route. Around 42 per cent in each group achieved the target of two lunchtime walks per week and the majority achieved one for the full eight weeks. By the end of the eight weeks there was a 10 per cent increase in participants who walked over 5000 steps and a 12 per cent decrease in participants who were walking fewer than 2500 steps. Even the small increase in number of steps is likely to contribute to enhancing health due to the positive relationship between physical activity and health (Tudor-Locke, 2010).

The fall in blood pressure following the eight weeks of walking was significantly greater in the natural setting than in the built group. This needs to be treated with caution, however, as the blood pressure in the built group was much lower at the start of the intervention. The blood pressure for the nature walking group only fell so that they had similar values to the built group at the end of the intervention. Any walk, whatever the environment, is useful for reducing blood pressure, especially if it slightly elevated prior to the start of a walking programme.

Other physiological measures taken (e.g. heart rate and autonomic control during rest, stressor, and recovery from a stressor) and evening cortisol measures, are indicative of levels of overall stress (Hellhammer et al., 2009). These were not different between the two groups. It may be the measures we took were not sensitive enough, or the stimulus of two walks (or less than that in some cases) was not enough to evoke these physiological responses. Other research exploring vascular markers (although not within the workplace) (Thompson et al., 2013) suggests that an eight-week green exercise intervention may be sufficient to evoke local vascular re-modelling changes. Thompson et al. (2013) analysed blood samples and identified changes in components utilised in building the extracellular matrix of the vascular walls following the intervention. It may indicate that local vascular changes are occurring, which matches the blood pressure changes that we saw in participants in the *Walks4work* study.

Our walks were self-led and had no facilitator input; although this represents a low-cost approach, it is likely this led to reduced adherence for some of the participants during the study period. On questioning participants at the completion of the study about walk leaders, participants overwhelmingly did not wish to have a walk leader from outside the company but to have a fellow employee promote the walks. Interestingly, those who had formed their own walk groups were still walking regularly when we visited the company two years later, showing a long-term behaviour change. Walk champions from within the company to assist in promoting the walks are essential for future interventions.

Although our *Walks4work* study found psychological changes including a reduction in perceived stress, future research into the effect of repeated exposure to green exercise is required in order to understand the potential role of lunchtime workplace green exercise interventions on modifying physical and mental health, particularly among highly stressed or hypertensive individuals. Detailed and rigorous studies are needed to explore the benefits and limitations. Additionally, it is essential that evaluation of any intervention is undertaken to use any findings as evidence for workplaces and for passing on good practice to other companies. Therefore, this should be supported by measures of fidelity by including adherence, exposure, quality of delivery and participant responsiveness/engagement.

For green exercise interventions to be successful there are potential barriers to overcome including perception of risks (such as safety) and the perception that there is a lack of time to undertake a walk. This may be facilitated by clear walking routes with an indication of the length of time of the walk. Walking with partners, groups and walk leaders (as mentioned above) may help alleviate some of these perceptions of risk and further engage more individuals and have the added benefit of social support that is so important for reducing stress. Additionally, an initial driver to engage a whole range of different individuals from different backgrounds would also be useful in altering social norms to elicit a behaviour change and change in culture within the company. Perhaps, most importantly, is to engage managers throughout the process and involve them in the promotion of green exercise. In our *Walks4work* study we found that where immediate line-managers were engaged in the intervention, participants were much more likely to complete the suggested walks. The economic analysis of the cost-effectiveness of green exercise interventions within workplaces needs to be undertaken, alongside providing clear evidence and guidance to help employers make calculated decisions about using green exercise initiatives within their own workplace.

Conclusions

The outdoor space close to a workplace can be a valuable asset to enhance employer and employee health and wellbeing. Many cultural, behavioural and planning factors, though, are required to facilitate its use. Green exercise helps increase levels of physical activity and provides a respite from stressful situations during a working day. Green exercise or viewing nature may be a useful positive coping mechanism to alter stress appraisal and elicit a positive behaviour change and reduce negative physiological and psychological changes. We conclude that green exercise at or near the workplace should be attractive to employees and employers alike as they offer a physical and mental wellbeing boost during the working day with very little investment. Unfortunately, many people are not engaging with green spaces around their workplace, mainly because of a perceived lack of time. A shift of culture and attitude within whole workplaces is required to facilitate the use of green exercise. If workplaces do engage with green exercise, we expect the employer will find a reduction in stress and fewer sick days with concurrent improvements in job performance and overall productivity.

Chapter 14

Green exercise and dementia

Neil Mapes

Introduction

Dementia has become a dominant narrative in my life. I was six years old when my 'little nan' Annie clearly started deteriorating in health. Parkinson's and then dementia led her to a bed in a cottage hospital in Essex, a frightening experience looking back at my younger self and seeing the grandmother I loved change so dramatically. My granddad Vic, Annie's husband, then went on to be diagnosed with Alzheimer's type Dementia. I recall him arriving outside our house in his old car with two watering cans already full of water from the well in his house: 'but Grandad we have water here at our house'. He proceeded happily to water the plants and was a man who spent many happy hours gardening and enjoying activity outdoors.

I share some of my personal family story here because it is important that from the start we remember and continue to remind ourselves that people with dementia are people – a diverse range of wonderful individuals many of whom have had a connection to nature, to the outdoors and to physical activity. My family has deep roots within rural farming communities in Essex, stretching back at least the last two hundred years: growing food and the physical activity associated with it on both small and large scales is in my blood. Over time I have learned that how we live our lives is by far the most important factor in whether we live healthily or not. It is also influential for avoiding illness or then coping when it does come into our lives. Right up until my grandfather's death he was collecting and chopping fire wood from the fields, to such an extent that he had literally 'shed-loads' of fire wood.

Dementia Adventure was set up after supporting Annie and Vic and my mother and subsequently hundreds of other families living with dementia stretching over two decades. The problem that we identified was rather simple: when dementia came into the life of an individual all too often that person was indoors too much of the time at a clear detriment to their physical health, emotional and social well-being. We simply wanted to get more people out of their rooms and buildings more of the time. We wanted to offer people more choices and more opportunities to get out into nature. Our mission is to enable people living with dementia to get outdoors, connect with nature, themselves and their community and retain a sense of adventure in their lives.

The complexities of the range of dementias are still to be fully understood, and whilst we wait for medical advances to bring news of cures, green exercise is arguably one of the most easily accessible evidence-based therapies in enabling people with dementia to have a life worth living. Not only is it free and accessible, we do not need to be taught or learn how to engage with it. In a time when many resources are directed to indoor multi-sensory environments to support well-being, we are at risk of forgetting about the original multi-sensory environment (the great outdoors). We will share here some of the evidence base outlining the role of green exercise for people living with dementia drawing on the Greening Dementia report (Clark et al., 2013) and more recent emerging evidence. We will also share some of our nature-based adventures which utilise a positive risk-taking approach and highlight how we can maintain our personal and emotional connection with nature through green exercise, despite having dementia. I firmly believe that regular green exercise can not only help prevent us getting dementia in the first place, but can also help slow down the progression of dementia and help alleviate or dampen the symptoms. Most of all, green exercise can be fun and if anyone might be needing more fun in their lives then surely that is people coming to terms with this thing we currently call dementia.

John Zeisel (2009) has observed: 'One of the biggest questions facing those living with dementia today is: should I take a pill or take a walk? There is little question that the answer is take a walk. Walking supports body and mind health and the sooner we start to exercise, the better will be our lives with dementia. Dementia Adventure is on the right path to living a quality life, even with dementia.'

The importance of green exercise for people living with dementia

In the UK, dementia directly affects around 800,000 people and a further 670,000 carers. For each of these individuals there is a unique personal family story and journey with dementia. The case for making progress with dementia as a societal issue has been well made with annual costs to the health service, local government and families currently estimated at £23 billion (Prince et al., 2014). With an ageing population the number of people living with dementia in the UK is predicted to double in the next 30 years. But this assumes no changes in behaviours and policies: I believe we can alter that projected statistic if we all look at how we can engage with people with dementia so that they can live life to the full.

There is currently no cure for any type of dementia; there are also no universally accepted, effective treatments for reversing the degenerative and chronic symptoms. In many cases, unpaid family carers deliver the bulk of care, often at a high cost to their own physical and mental health. However, there is hope with new medical and scientific treatments on the horizon and there are existing medications, services and methods of support that can help people with dementia to live well right now. Although in recent years there have been significant developments in government policy on dementia, most notably with a focus on 'dementia-friendly communities', none are explicitly focused on outdoor activities and green spaces. Parks, allotments, rivers, canals and waterways, coastal areas and mountainous wilder spaces are all natural environments in which we individually and collectively belong, celebrate, exercise and relax.

In our experience, too many people living with dementia are subtly and overtly prevented from getting outdoors at all and when they are supported to do so it is a means to an end (i.e. travelling from one inside space to another inside space (and service) resulting in an unnecessary subsequent decline in well-being). Natural England is committed to increasing the number and range of people who can experience and benefit from access to the natural environment, and through the 'Outdoors for All Programme' is leading the government's ambition that *'everyone should have fair access to a good quality natural environment'*. In recent years Natural England have taken a stance on supporting people with dementia to benefit from the outdoors and now organisations across the board, including those which manage green spaces and whose primary focus is conservation, are beginning to look at what they can do to become more accessible and supportive of people living with dementia (Clark et al., 2013).

Yet the local services and projects which currently exist specifically to bring the benefits of green exercise to more people with dementia are fragmented and often have a qualitative focus due to the nature of delivering the projects and have not been resourced to robustly evaluate the impact of the outdoor programmes. This issue was recently highlighted by Public Health England in identifying local physical inactivity interventions (Public Health England, 2015). Specifically with regards to dementia the recently updated Cochrane review on exercise programmes for people with dementia showed promising results for improving activities of daily living (only) but also concluded that additional well-designed trials are needed in this area to investigate the best types of exercise programmes for people with different types of and stages of dementia (Forbes et al., 2015). Therefore, we should continue, with caution, reminding ourselves that there is unlikely to be a 'one-size fits all' approach to solutions for people with dementia.

We now know that engagement with the natural environment can have a positive effect on people living with dementia (Clark et al., 2013). The benefits can be broadly themed into physical, emotional and social benefits, and comprise: i) better eating and sleeping patterns, better fitness and mobility and fewer falls; ii) improved emotional state through reduced stress, agitation, anger, apathy and depression; and iii) improved sense of well-being, self-esteem and control leading to improved social interaction and a sense of belonging. But what we do now need is more robust larger scale research into the benefits of different activities for different groups of people with dementia. It will thus be important to increase the scale and offering of physical activity programmes so that more people living with dementia can access and enjoy them.

A central public health message many people in our societies seem to have understood is that by adopting healthier behaviours such as stopping smoking, exercising regularly and living healthier lives we reduce our risk of heart disease (and other conditions), but the message that these lifestyle changes can also help reduce our risk of getting dementia has not yet been heard by the general public. Of all the modifiable lifestyle factors which have been studied in relation to reducing the risk of getting dementia, exercise consistently comes out as the most effective way to reduce risk. A number of significant research projects have highlighted this evidence in the last few years but perhaps Peter Elwood summarised it best in an Alzheimer's Society (2013) article:

> The size of reduction in the instance of disease owing to these simple healthy steps has really amazed us and is of enormous importance in an aging population…What the research shows is that following a healthy lifestyle confers surprisingly large benefits to health – healthy behaviours have a far more beneficial effect than any medical treatment or preventative procedure.

For the 800,000 people in the UK currently with a diagnosis of dementia, there remains much hope that green exercise can not only support happier healthier lives but can also contribute to slowing down the progression of the disease (Mapes and Hine, 2011; Brewin, 2015; Cook, 2015).

Nature-based adventures facilitate positive risk-taking

Our adventure provision at Dementia Adventure takes a variety of forms, and is centrally concerned with supporting people to share and enjoy activity together in nature. Underpinning everything we do is a positive risk-taking approach, which is grounded in the concept of risk/benefit assessment. We believe that anything is possible if we thoroughly examine and plan for the risks and benefits associated with an activity. Our work at Dementia Adventure operates at three levels. First we aim to get people active, enjoying exercise out in nature; second, if we cannot do that, we simply aim to get people out of buildings into nature (even if only for five minutes); and third we bring nature into buildings into the lives of people who may spend all of their day indoors. The sheer variety and endless ways of connecting with nature means that we can support individuals to engage with activities that might feel risky and give them a sense of living and are personalised to them, whether it is sitting listening to the birds in the park or white-water rafting.

We have designed and led a variety of nature-based adventures since establishing Dementia Adventure in 2009. These adventures include dementia-friendly walks, woodland celebration days, and bespoke group adventure holidays such as walking in the Lakes, sailing, and white-water rafting. All these have implications for designers and planners, who have a role to play in making green spaces and green exercise accessible, safe and enjoyable for people living with dementia.

Our provision is carefully designed and researched. People living with dementia and their family carers often generate the original idea for the adventures and are consulted in how to deliver the adventure as well as reviewing its impact and success. We have specialist insurance cover, support people to access specialist personal travel insurance and have developed a successful model of adventure provision. This model ensures there are more people on the adventure 'without dementia' than there are with dementia. The model also includes issuing a special invitation and motivation to get out into nature, a personalised experience with choices on the adventure and creating a 'dementia-friendly' environment. A typical adventure holiday will involve twelve people, four people living with dementia, four family carers and four staff or volunteers. People who are further down the road in their dementia journey, many of whom are living in care homes, have also benefitted from our park walks and woodland days out.

Walking in nature and dementia

Walking has many physical and mental health benefits and helps us to maintain social connections while being in communities and nature. The Chief Medical Officer recommends that adults should undertake at least 30 minutes of moderate-intensity physical activity, such as brisk walking, on five or more days a week (Department of Health, 2011b). Regular walking, as part of a healthy lifestyle, helps reduce the risk of a variety of conditions including cardiovascular disease, strokes, arthritis, anxiety and stress. Recent research from the USA shows that moderate but regular exercise boosts the size of the parts of the brain that shrink with age; exercise promotes the growth of new cells in the brain and improves cell and tissue repair mechanisms. For those who already have dementia, it can help slow down progression of the disease (Erickson et al., 2012). Leading personalities in the dementia sector are now working to ensure that the benefits of green exercise are applied to people living with dementia.

> It is likely that the need for contact with the natural environment and the feelings we have about nature and being outdoors are hardwired, partly because this is a source of food. Sunshine, flowers, shade, moonlight and trees are all so much a part of our basic nature that no one has to be taught to respond appropriately to such stimuli. Again not surprisingly, gardens and nature are much appreciated by those with the illness.
>
> (Zeisel, 2009)

> Nature is sometimes taken for granted and undervalued. But people cannot flourish without the benefits and services our natural environment provides. Nature is a complex, interconnected system. A healthy, properly functioning natural environment is the foundation of sustained economic growth, prospering communities and personal well-being.
>
> (HM Government, 2011)

Dementia-friendly walks

Parks and publicly-accessible green open spaces are often close to home. Dementia Adventure has delivered supported and inclusive walks for people living with dementia since 2010. We have also helped create and sustain a wide variety of dementia-friendly walks around the country. Participants include people living in their own homes, who often simply want to walk as much as they can, as well as people living with dementia in care homes with more advanced stages of dementia who are at risk from being separated from nature and from wider society. In 2014 we expanded our provision from its base in Chelmsford to include walks in Redbridge, Barking and Dagenham, Stroud and in a variety of locations across Leicester. We have done this by identifying local partners and lead individuals and providing them with a comprehensive two-day dementia-friendly walk leader training course. This course supports people with the resources to be confident to deliver a series of walks specifically for people living with dementia. During 2015, nearly 900 people enjoyed activity on a dementia-friendly walk with partner organisations delivering these experiences ranging from local authorities to Age UK organisations. People living with dementia have said:

I like to walk as much is allowed.

I had a good day.

I had the best ice cream.

This is the best day.

Walks are a lot of fun.

Care home staff commented:

These walks have enhanced the lives of our residents immensely, enabling them to experience being in a different environment, and also to socialise with others living with the various stages of dementia. It was also good for our staff members to chat with care staff from other homes, to gain ideas and also learn of their experiences. It has been so rewarding for care staff and family to see the pleasure it has given our residents.

We don't usually get much response from the resident but he seemed to come alive on this visit.

One resident said he had an overwhelming feeling of camaraderie, a sense of belonging.

A resident was able to identify trees and flowers. I didn't know what they were.

It was nice for the residents to be with so many people.

Family carers were able to enjoy the visit without the stress of having to look after their loved one.

Family carers have said:

You could see the residents were enjoying it.

It was mum as I always knew her; I had her back with me again.

I'd like to do more visits of this kind.

A park walk partner organisation observed:

We had a new lady come down last week (she lost her husband a month ago and has been very distant since) she was adamant that she didn't like anything and didn't want to walk and so on, but she did walk last week and spotted a toothless park keeper that made her laugh very much. She returned this week with her carer and her carer said that she had been laughing about the toothless park keeper all week. And so she came back and walked again and they hope to continue joining us every week.

Woodland celebration days

Dementia Adventure has worked with the VisitWoods team at the Woodland Trust on a succession of projects. One of these in 2012 was our woodland celebration day: Dementia Adventure convened 77 people, including 38 people living with dementia, for a day of activity at Lochore Meadows in Scotland. The day was blessed with sunshine. Participants came from a variety of backgrounds and included family members and carers from residential and nursing homes as well as active younger groups of people living with dementia. A variety of nature activities were on offer for people with different interests, varying levels of need and ability. People living with dementia using wheelchairs enjoyed the picnic lunch, views across the lake, and reminisced about the location and elements of nature from their younger days. Some of the participants remembered the coal mine which stood on the site before the planting of the woodland, whilst others reminisced about family days out enjoyed as children. Indoor activities were also on offer for people to make nature collages with the materials they collected outdoors. The more physically able participants enjoyed these activities as well as a loch side walk with a small group taking an extended walk around the woodland.

We gave participants of the celebration day strips of cotton to record their connections with nature. These were tied to trees and bushes along the loch walk and included the following reflections on the importance of outdoor activity:

Seeing the natural scenery and different types of plants.

Animal sounds, people laughing, children singing.

I loved feeling the sun on my skin for the first time in ages.

Beauty of the country and wildlife.

I enjoyed being in the fresh air.

Meeting up with other people and walking together.

I loved smelling the flowers.

I enjoyed looking over the loch.

People are so friendly.

This woodland celebration day was intentionally created and designed in the format of a family day out, albeit an extended family of nearly 80 people. Integral to this experience was a picnic lunch, which made everyone feel more at home and which triggered memories for some of childhood picnics and fun outdoors.

In 2014, Hampshire Council worked with Dementia Adventure to design and deliver a farm-based adventure. This is an example of how mutual benefit can be gained by integrating health and social care with green space providers. Dementia Adventure ran a three-day experiential programme called 'Home Outdoors' to bring together parks and care home staff. The first training day supported them to work together to design and deliver an outdoors adventure which took place at Manor Farm Country Park. We then brought the successfully integrated team back together for day 3 to look at the wide variety of opportunities for co-produced adventures with local people involving other green spaces. We continue to work with organisations in Hampshire supporting a range of Dementia-friendly outdoor activities in parks as well as care farms.

Dementia-friendly green spaces

Through our work with an increasing number of green space and conservation organisations, we have learnt that with the right commitment and approach, many can enable more people with dementia to enjoy activity outdoors. Dementia-friendly green spaces are welcoming, easy to access, easy to find your way around and there is information about what you can see, hear, touch, smell and taste. A dementia-friendly green space has staff and volunteers who are aware of dementia and can offer specific support if needed in a way which is respectful and they adopt a risk-benefit approach in providing a stimulating yet safe environment.

By beginning to look at our green spaces through the lens of dementia we have also learned how difficult it can be for some people simply to get to and get around a green space. By designing these spaces more effectively people will be enabled to self-lead outdoor activity such as walking. In addition there will always be people who need more information, more support and sometimes dementia-specific groups in order to enjoy some green exercise in these locations. We have found that staff and volunteers working in a range of organisations are increasingly aware of dementia because of the profile it has received in the media and because of the increasing numbers of people living with the condition. These people want to play their role in helping people to live well with dementia but often lack some knowledge, confidence or experience in effectively engaging and including people with dementia to enjoy green space and the outdoors.

Dementia Adventure is working to bring together green space organisations with health and social care organisations who directly support people living with dementia to solve respective problems and work together for mutual benefit, all around the theme of activity outdoors. During 2015 Dementia Adventure has been leading a national partnership project called DEN (Dementia and Engagement with Nature), which has consulted people living with dementia about their activity and engagement with nature and the outdoors. The aim of the DEN project was to gather the views of people living with dementia and carers about the role of outdoor activity and natural outdoor spaces in helping people with dementia to live well. The key themes from the research included the importance of activities such as walking (both informal and guided), wildlife activities and the importance of places such as parks and gardens and the presence of water. Dementia Adventure is now working with Natural England and other national and local organisations to implement a national movement of green exercise programmes specifically for people living with dementia, informed by the DEN project and the Greening Dementia research (Clark et al., 2013).

Dementia Adventure holidays and short breaks

Dementia Adventure has designed and led a variety of bespoke residential holidays since 2011 including walking in the Lake District and Devon, Take Five breaks on the Isle of Wight and Isle of Man, canal boat holidays, and sailing and white-water rafting holidays. Here is a selection of comments from our participants on the holidays:

> Wonderful way to have a supported holiday in a beautiful location with friendly helpful staff.

The first time I have been able to relax so much in years.

Challenging, enjoyable, worthwhile, good experience (amazing), an excellent break, brilliant company and very supportive staff.

Although the memory may fade Dennis certainly seemed invigorated and satisfied with the holiday and mixed group.

These include hands-on sailing holidays provided in Cornwall in partnership with Classic Sailing and in Essex in partnership with the Sea Change Sailing Trust. John was only 54 when he came on the voyage on the Eve of St Mawes in Cornwall with his wife Annie. They both had a marvellous time – John said at the end of the first day – 'I've enjoyed myself, everyone's been happy – no arguments! – It's a good day, isn't it?' – and at the end of the second day he said 'We've had such a laugh, and it's cheered me up no end – It's nice to know that there are some very, very kind people out there – they are looking after us.' The sailing adventures involve people living with dementia supported by someone who knows them well actively crewing the boat, steering a course, pulling ropes and sharing the challenge of sailing from one location to another over a three- or five-day sail.

Tony is living with dementia and took part in the Essex sailing holiday. He was part of the crew which successfully sailed 92 nautical miles during their group holiday, and said:

I never thought I would have such a chance and I have learnt so much from being on deck with the experienced crew. The sailing was excellent – it was all great.

Sam and Ben (his sons) said:

What a week and what a team! It was brilliant to meet everyone, to see the beautiful river estuaries, to survive a day of rough seas and high winds, to keep laughing and to learn about the boat and its history. Above all it was so good to see Dad joining in and gaining confidence day by day.

Christopher (living with dementia) said:

It was a great experience which others should do… it was fun and the people were charming, and the food was good!

Other feedback from family members included:

He has been very positive since coming back from the trip: more positive and animated and with it. Thank you.

Conclusions

People living with dementia face many challenges during their life journey. At each step of this journey green exercise presents opportunities for maintaining and improving lives. It presents opportunities to maintain connections with the people and places we love, to enjoy purposeful activity which is good for our well-being, which can be sensitively tailored to our personal and cultural needs. Participating in green exercise can also enable people to thrive instead of simply survive. We have highlighted our adventures to show how dementia-friendly walks, woodland experiences and holidays are beneficial forms of green exercise for people living with dementia: all have illustrated the importance of opening horizons and expanding boundaries for everyone in our communities.

Chapter 15

The benefits of greener and healthier economies

Jules Pretty and Jo Barton

From material consumption to consumption of nature

It has long been assumed that increased material consumption and rising per capita gross domestic product (GDP) inevitably leads to increased wellbeing. We now know this is not true. The GDP:wellbeing gap has been partly caused by the negative environmental and health externalities of material consumption. Pollution causes harm, costs money to clean up, but appears on the positive side of the balance sheet for economic growth. Over-consumption of food contributes to GDP, but can cause obesity, which in turn costs to treat, again appearing to contribute to measures of GDP.

We have proposed a model to characterise how behaviour affects the choices and behaviours of individuals (Figure 15.1). It is widely assumed that *material*

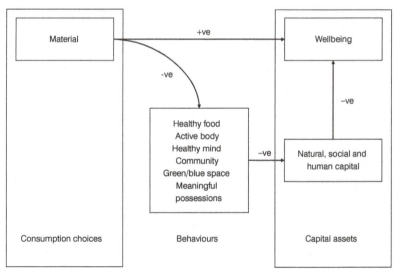

Figure 15.1 The side-effects of material consumption of goods and services and impacts on wellbeing

consumption (MC) positively affects wellbeing. However, this same MC produces negative side-effects that influence six factors critical for health and wellbeing (Layard, 2006; Jackson, 2009; NEA, 2011; NEF, 2013; Pretty, 2013: Pretty et al., 2015): i) healthy food; ii) active body; iii) healthy mind; iv) links with community and family; v) contact with nature and green/blue space; and vi) attachment to meaningful possessions. As each of these is negatively affected, either separately or in combination, so natural, social and human capital are eroded, and wellbeing itself declines.

Figure 15.2 proposes a variant whereby *environmentally sustainable consumption* (ESC) substitutes for MC, thus improving wellbeing and stocks of renewable natural, social and human capital assets, and *sustainable behaviours involving non-material consumption* (SBs-NMC) are substituted and sustained. SBs-NMC includes activities in nature (e.g. gardening, angling, walking) and in communities (e.g. volunteering, sports, meetings, community ceremonies and rituals). These are known to have direct benefits for individual wellbeing of both donors and recipients (NEF, 2013).

Thus increases in environmentally sustainable consumption and sustainable behaviours that substitute for material consumption result in behaviours that build capital assets and improve wellbeing, whilst at the same time slowing the convergence of consumption patterns towards high and unsustainable levels that threaten the integrity of planetary natural capital (Anderson and Bows, 2011; Pretty, 2013; Costanza et al., 2014). Some negative movements have often been accompanied by positive progress (away from costs and towards benefits). For example, there is evidence in some affluent countries of more social isolation and loneliness brought

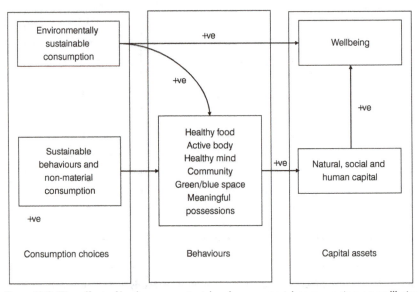

Figure 15.2 The effect of both green material and non-material consumption on wellbeing

about by changing family and community structures, yet at the same time the rise in social media has increased online social connections. As the obesity crisis emerged, so has grown an interest in the sustainability of food and agriculture.

Aggregated together, the benefits of material consumption and the counter-trends should have delivered considerable improvements to aggregate wellbeing. Yet, measured as life satisfaction at the population level, they have not. At the global level, the iron cage of arithmetic is stark: increasing convergence by poorer and developing countries on patterns of high material consumption typically prevalent in affluent countries will put further pressure on global natural capital (Pretty, 2013). Substitution of material consumption by both environmentally sustainable consumption and sustainable behaviours is becoming increasingly urgent, implying the need for green technology development and widespread behaviour change, supported by policies, new forms of social organisation and regulations that incentivise rapid uptake.

The evidence for successful interventions is, however, limited: more often than not advances towards environmentally sustainable consumption (e.g. more sustainable agriculture, greater energy efficiency in industrial processes, greater renewable energy production, increased material recycling and reuse, adoption of non-ozone damaging refrigerants) has been overtaken by increases in the number of people consuming and their expanding levels of consumption. In affluent countries, some policies and regulations have shifted individual behaviours towards greater wellbeing, but generally these again have been limited in number (e.g. shift to non-leaded petrol, restrictions on public and private locations where smoking is permitted), or affect only small subsets of the population (e.g. recommendations for physical activity, daily consumption of fruit and vegetables).

Creating economic benefits

The UK Office for National Statistics (2013) is now measuring wellbeing at the national level in the UK; but these measures have not yet changed policy or practice, particularly in health and social care. Mitchell and Popham (2008) concluded that 'environments that promote good health might be crucial in the fight to reduce health inequalities'. There is growing evidence showing that choices and behaviours at the individual level can make significant contributions to wellbeing, regardless of technological and policy progress to support shifts from material consumption to environmentally sustainable consumption. Such activities that result in greater wellbeing, substitute for material consumption, and result in benefits for natural capital and social capital include gardening, walking and running, nature watching and visiting, spiritual contemplation and social prayer, fishing, organised sports, volunteering, joining societies and clubs, playing music, engaging in art and writing.

This suggests a key dilemma: reducing material consumption to save the planet undermines an economy founded on continuing consumption; yet continuing material consumption at current rates to sustain the economy destroys the planet.

Yet a substantial financial dividend could be released by a greener and healthier economy (Beatley and Newman, 2013) centred on healthy food, regular engagement with nature, regular physical activity, the use of the power of thought and contemplation, the enhancement of social bonds, and increased attachment to possessions and places. Table 15.1 summarises the costs of the health externalities arising from modern lifestyles in the UK. The annual direct cost of mental ill-health, dementias, obesity, physical inactivity, diabetes, loneliness and cardio-vascular disease (including strokes) is £82 billion; the full cost to the whole economy is approximately £250 billion annually (18.6 per cent of GDP). The revenue expenditure of the 248 national health system (NHS) Trusts in 2011–2012 was £102 billion.

There are many possible interactions between causes and outcomes. Mental ill-health will have direct costs and consequences; it may also lead to reductions in physical activity, which in turn could influence caloric intake. Loneliness could have an impact on onset of dementias. The individual costs of each of the seven conditions in Table 15.1 thus will include some of the costs for treatment for other conditions. Nonetheless, some costs have been allocated according to the presentation of a condition to the health service (e.g. CVD, diabetes), and these are real costs to the service providers. Others costs, such as of loneliness, are calculated from combinations of drivers. We thus assume a cautious reduction of costs by 25 per cent to account for interactive effects and co-morbidities.

This implies there are health savings to be made if prevalence of these conditions and recruitment to medical treatment is reduced or prevented. Upstream activities and behaviours that prevent these negative health externalities improve the wellbeing of individuals and result in reduced costs to both the health service and economy at large. The Chief Medical Officer (CMO, 2013) suggests that the health costs of lifestyles and behaviours comprise a new canon for prevention. With an ageing population, cost inflation, and pressures on revenue, the UK's National Health Service as a system needs to find ways to invest in prevention rather than wait until it has to treat conditions. Table 15.1 shows that the annual health and social costs per individual, and thus the savings for each avoided condition, vary between £500 and £12,000, though are higher for dementias.

The cost of a single in-patient stay for an obese person is £3215; the average cost per Accident and Emergency presentation is £108; the average cost of a CVD hospital admission £4614 (NHS Reference Costs, 2015). The benefits to the national health system of programmes that prevent recruitment are thus relatively small per person, but aggregated up very quickly at population level, suggesting that investments in healthy lifestyle programmes would bring many benefits. Befriending programmes for the elderly-lonely reduce the annual number of general practitioner visits from 10.8 to 6.7, saving £195 per person; walking for health programmes produce £623 of benefits per person annually; mentally-ill patients accessing CBT and chronic disease management save £2000 per person.

The Chief Medical Officer (2013) estimates that there is a 6–10 per cent annual rate of return on investments made in early life interventions. The costs

Table 15.1 The costs of the health externalities arising from modern lifestyles in the UK

Condition	Proportion of population affected	Number affected	Annual cost to NHS (£billion)	Full annual cost to economy (£billion)	Annual NHS cost per person with condition (£)	Full annual cost per person per condition (£)
Mental ill-health	17.6 % of adults 10% of children	8.8 million	21.0	105.0	2,390	11,900
Dementias	13% of >65 year olds	0.75 million	20.0	20.0	26,700	nd
Obesity[1]	26% of adults 15% of children	13 million adults 1.9 million children	5.0	20.0	384	1,538
Physical inactivity[2]	20% of adults completely inactive	10 million adults	1.8	8.2	nd	nd
Diabetes (type 2)	4.5% of adults	2.9 million	13.75	29.0	4,741	10,000
Loneliness	30% of >65 year olds	0.9 million	10.0	40.0	768	3,072
Cardio-vascular disease (including hypertension and strokes)		1.84 million in-patient episodes (of which 0.24 million for strokes): 180,000 deaths	10.5 (of which 1.8 for strokes)	22.6	5,437–7,500	11,812
Total (assuming all costs independent and additive)			82.1	244.8		
Total costs (assuming one quarter of costs double-counted)			61.5	183.6		

Notes: 1 Obesity costs are assumed to be the same for adults and children. The annual health costs of obesity in the USA are $147 billion, equivalent to $1,429 per treated person (CDC, 2014). 2 The individual costs of physical inactivity are not calculated as most are manifested in other co-morbidities (e.g. obesity, diabetes). Source: Pretty et al. (2015)

of one year in a children's residential home are £149,000, of one admission to inpatient mental health services £25,000; the long-term costs of child obesity are approximately £600 million, the annual short-term costs of emotional, conduct and hyperkinetic disorders in children some £1.5 billion. Half of all adult mental illness begins before the age of 15, and 75 per cent before the age of 18 (Foresight, 2008; CMO, 2013). Mental health problems track into adulthood, just as being overweight and obesity do (Knapp et al., 2011).

In the USA, the Union of Concerned Scientists (2014) has indicated that one-third (750,000 people) of annual fatalities are attributable to cardio-vascular disease, causing direct annual medical costs of $273 billion. The average American consumes just 0.8 portions of fruit and 1.6 portions of vegetables daily (USDA ERS, 2013); each additional daily fruit and vegetable portion reduces the risk of stroke and heart disease by 4-5 per cent (Dauchet et al., 2006). One additional portion consumed daily would prevent 30,000 deaths; consumption at recommended levels would prevent 127,000 deaths (calculated to have $11 trillion of present value arising from longevity and better lives).

The UK government's public health strategy, *Healthy Lives, Healthy People* (DoH, 2011), explicitly recognises that health considerations are an important part of planning policy. The National Planning Policy Framework (DCLG, 2012) further makes it clear that local planning authorities have a responsibility to promote healthy communities, and a number of local authorities have drawn up supplementary planning documents (SPDs) that seek to limit the number of fast food outlets in close proximity to schools. The challenge is to create a built environment that is 'sociable and green' (O'Donnell et al., 2014). The UK Public Services (Social Value Act) 2012 'requires public authorities to have regard to economic, social and environmental wellbeing'.

A greener economy that emphasises ecological public health (Frumkin, 2005; Lang and Rayner, 2012) would be one in which attention is paid to the environmental and social context of the public not yet ill, patients and all professionals and families engaged in treatment and care (Pencheon, 2012; CMO, 2013). The Marmot Review (2008) of health inequalities concluded that 'economic growth is not the most important measure of our country's success', and prioritised the accumulation of the positive effects on wellbeing across the whole life course by building social capital, encouraging active travel, use of public transport, availability of green space and healthy eating, and promotion of nature-based interventions for health. Public Health England (2013a, b) has observed that there is a need to find ways 'to walk out of necessity', not choice. Some structures and policies are being established: the challenge of widespread adherence to behaviour change remains, as does the wider narrative about the benefits of greener and prosocial economies.

As environmental and social context influences wellbeing and health, positive policies to shape economies and societies for individuals will increase the likelihood that more people will be able to live their lives well and for longer. A greener, healthier economy would prioritise choices for both environmentally sustainable consumption and sustainable behaviours involving green exercise

Bibliography

Adamo, K. B., Sheel, A. W., Onywera, V., Waudo, J., Boit, M. and Tremblay, M. S. (2012). Child obesity and fitness levels among Kenyan and Canadian children from urban and rural environments: A KIDS-CAN Research Alliance study. *International Journal of Pediatric Obesity*, 6: 225–232.

Ader, R. and Cohen, N. (2002). Behaviorally conditional immunosuppression and murine systemic *lupus erythematosis*. *Science*, 215: 1534–36.

Ainsworth, M. D. S., Bell, S. M. and Stayton, D. J. (1974). Infant–mother attachment and social development. In Richards, M. P. M. (ed.), *The Integration of a Child into a Social World*. Cambridge: Cambridge University Press.

Ainsworth, B. E., Haskell, W. L., Herrmann, S. D., Meckes, N., Bassett, D. R., et al. (2011). 2011 compendium of physical activities: a second update of codes and MET values. *Medicine and Science in Sports and Exercise*, 43(8): 1575–1581.

Aked, J. and Thompson, S. (2011). *Five Ways to Wellbeing, New Applications, New Ways of Thinking*. London: New Economics Foundation.

Akers, A., Barton, J., Cossey, R., Gainsford, P., Griffin, M. and Micklewright, D. (2012). Visual color perception in green exercise: positive effects on mood and perceived exertion. *Environmental Science and Technology*, 46(16): 8661–8666.

Albrecht, G A. (2005). Solastalgia: a new concept in human health and identity. *PAN (Philosophy, Activism, Nature)*, 3: 41–55.

All Party Commission on Physical Activity (2014). *Tackling Physical Inactivity – a Coordinated Approach*. All Party Commission on Physical Activity.

Allen, J. and Balfour, R. (2014). *Natural Solutions for Tackling Health Inequalities*. London: Natural England.

Al-Nuaim, A. A., Al-Nakeeb, Y., Lyons, M., Al-Hazzaa, H., Nevill, A., et al. (2012). The prevalence of physical activity and sedentary behaviours relative to obesity among adolescents from Al-Ahsa, Saudi Arabia: Rural versus Urban variations. *Journal of Nutrition and Metabolism*, doi: 10.1155/2012/417589.

Altshuler, B. (1981). Modeling of dose-response relationships. *Environmental Health Perspectives*, 42: 23-27.

Alzheimer's Society (2013). *Research Findings show Exercise Plays Significant Role in Reducing Risk of Dementia*, Online at: www.alzheimers.org.uk/site/scripts/news_article.php?newsID=1896

Ambrose-Oji. B. (2010). *Forestry Commission Working with Civil Society*. Farnham: Forest Research.

Ambrose-Oji. B. (2013). *Mindfulness Practice in Woods and Forests: An Evidence Review*. Research Report for The Mersey Forest, Farnham: Forest Research.

Anderson, K. and Bows, A. (2011). Beyond 'dangerous' climate change: emission scenarios for a new world. *Philosophical Transcripts of the Royal Society* A, 369: 20–44.

Angkurawaranon, C., Wattanatchariya, N., Doyle, P. and Nitsch, D. (2013). Urbanization and non-communicable disease mortality in Thailand: an ecological correlation study. *Tropical Medicine and International Health*, 18: 130–40.

Annerstedt, M. and Wahrborg, P. (2011). Nature-assisted therapy: Systematic review of controlled and observational studies. *Scandinavian Journal of Public Health*, 39: 371–388.

Antonovsky, A. (1996). The salutogenic model as a theory to guide health promotion. *Health Promotion International*, 11: 11–18.

Arkenford (2013). *Watersports Participation Survey 2013. Executive Summary*. Online at: www.rya.org.uk/SiteCollectionDocuments/sportsdevelopment/Watersports_survey_Market_Review_2013_Executive_Summary_.pdf

Aronsson, J., Tighe, M. and Waite, S. (2014). *Woodland Health for Youth (WHY): An Evaluation of Physical Health Benefits Derived from Outdoor Learning in Natural Environments (LINE) for school-Age Children*. End of grant report. Plymouth: Plymouth University.

Asfeldt, M. and Hvenegaard, G. (2014). Perceived learning, critical elements and lasting impacts on university-based wilderness educational expeditions. *Journal of Adventure Education and Outdoor Learning*, 14: 132–152.

Ashbullby, K. J., Pahl, S., Webley, P. and White, M. P. (2013). The beach as a setting for families' health promotion: A qualitative study with parents and children living in coastal regions in Southwest England. *Health and Place*, 23: 138–147.

Asher, S. R. and Paquette, J. A. (2003). Loneliness and peer relations in childhood. *Current Directions in Psychological Science*, 12 (3): 75–78.

Aspinall, P., Mavros, P., Coyne, R. and Roe, J. (2013). The urban brain: analysing outdoor physical activity with mobile EEG. *British Journal of Sports Medicine*, 1: 1–6.

Astell-Burt, T., Feng, X. and Kolt, G. S. (2013a). Greener neighborhoods, slimmer people? Evidence from 246,920 Australians. *International Journal of Obesity*, doi: 10.1038/ijo.2013.64.

Astell-Burt, T., Feng, X. and Kolt, G. S. (2013b). Mental health benefits of neighbourhood green space are stronger among physically active adults in middle-to-older age: Evidence from 260,061 Australians. *Preventive Medicine*, 57: 601–606.

Australian Bureau of Statistics (2008). *National Survey of Mental Health and Wellbeing: Summary of Results, 2007*, Canberra: ABS.

Australian Bureau of Statistics (2012). *Gender Indicators, Australia, 2012*, Canberra: ABS.

Australian Bureau of Statistics (2013). *Population Projections, Australia, 2012 (base) to 2101*, Canberra: ABS.

Australian Bureau of Statistics (2014). *Regional Population Growth, Australia 2012–2013*, Canberra: ABS.

Australian Institute of Health and Welfare (2013). Overweight and obesity. Online at: www.aihw.gov.au/overweight-and-obesity/

Baird, B., Smallwood, J. and Schooler, J. W. (2011). Back to the future: autobiographical planning and the functionality of mind-wandering. *Consciousness and Cognition*, 20(4): 1604–1611.

Bandura, A. (1977). Self-efficacy: toward a unifying theory of behavioral change. *Psychological Review*, 84: 191.

Barton, J. and Pretty, J. (2010). What is the best dose of nature and green exercise for improving mental health? A multi-study analysis. *Environmental Science and Technology*, 44: 3947–3955.

Barton, J., Hine, R. E. and Pretty, J. (2009). The health benefits of walking in greenspaces of high natural and heritage value. *Journal of Integrative Environmental Science*, 6(4): 261–278.

Barton, J., Hine, R. E. and Pretty, J. (2010). *The TurnAround Project – Phase 2: Follow on from the TurnAround 2007 Project – Phase 1*. Report for the Wilderness Foundation. Colchester: University of Essex.

Barton, J., Griffin, M. and Pretty, J. (2012). Exercise-, nature- and socially interactive-based initiatives improve mood and self-esteem in the clinical population. *Perspectives in Public Health*, 132: 89–96.

Barton, J., Sandercock, G., Pretty, J. and Wood, C. (2014). The effect of playground- and nature-based playtime interventions on physical activity and self-esteem in UK school children. *International Journal of Environmental Health Research*, 12: 1–11.

Barts Health NHS Trust (2013). TLC research summary. Online at: www.sduhealth.org.uk/news-events/news/214/Barts-Health-NHS-Trust-saves-100000-with-a-bit-of-TLC

Bateson, G. (1972). *Steps to an Ecology of the Mind*. New York: Ballantine Books.

Bathrellou, E., Lazarou, C., Panagiotakos, D. B. and Sidossis, L. S. (2007). Physical activity patterns and sedentary behaviours of children from urban and rural areas of Cyprus. *Central European Journal of Public Health*, 15: 66–70.

Bauman, A., Smith, B., Stoker, L., Bellew, B. and Booth, M. (1999). Geographical influences upon physical activity participation: evidence of a 'coastal effect'. *Australian and New Zealand Journal of Public Health*, 23: 322–324.

Bauman, A. E., Reis, R. S., Sallis, J. F., Wells, J. C., Loos, R. J. F. and Martin, B. W. (2012). Correlates of physical activity: why are some people physically active and others not? *The Lancet*, 380(9383): 258–271.

Beames, S. and Ross, H. (2010). Journeys outside the classroom. *Journal of Adventure Education and Outdoor Learning*, 10(2): 95–109.

Beatley, T. and Newman, P. (2013). Biophilic cities are sustainable, resilient cities. *Sustainability* 5, 3328–3345.

Beil, K. and Hanes, D. (2013). The influence of urban natural and built environments on physiological and psychological measures of stress: A pilot study. *International Journal of Environmental Research and Public Health*, 10: 1250–1267.

Belk, R. W. (1988). Possessions and the extended self. *Journal of Consumer Research*, 15(2): 139–168.

Belk, R. W. (1991). Possessions and the sense of the past. In Belk, R. W. (ed.), *Highways and Buyways.*, Duluth, MN: Association for Consumer Research.

Bell, M. M. (1997). The ghosts of place. *Theory and Society*, 26: 813–836.

Benson, H., Dusek, J. A., Sherwood, J. B., Lam, P., Bethea, C. F., et al. (2006). Study of the therapeutic effects of intercessory prayer (STEP) in cardiac bypass patients. *American Heart Journal*, 151(4): 934–942.

Bentsen, P. (2013). Udeskole in Scandinavia: Teaching and learning in natural places. The New Nature Movement. Online at: www.childrenandnature.org/blog/2013/02/12/udeskole-in-scandinavia-teaching-learning-in-natural-places/

Bentsen, P. and Jensen, F. S. (2012). The nature of Udeskole: Outdoor learning theory and practice in Danish schools. *Journal of Adventure Education and Outdoor Learning*, 12(3): 199–219.

Berget, B., Ekeberg, Ø. and Braastad, B. (2008). Animal-assisted therapy with farm animals for persons with psychiatric disorders: Effects on self-efficacy, coping ability and quality of life, a randomized controlled trial. *Clinical Practice and Epidemiology in Mental Health*, 4: 9, doi: 10.1186/1745-0179-4-9.

Berget, B., Ekeberg, Ø., Pedersen, I. and Braastad, B. (2011). Animal-assisted therapy with farm animals for persons with psychiatric disorders: Effects on anxiety and depression, a randomized controlled trial. *Occupational Therapy in Mental Health*, 27: 50–64.

Berliner, D. (2011). Rational responses to high stakes testing: the case of curriculum narrowing and the harm that follows. *Cambridge Journal of Education*, 41(3): 287–302.

Berman, M. C., Jonides, J. and Kaplan, S. (2008). The cognitive benefits of interacting with nature. *Psychological Science*, 19: 1207–1212.

Berman, M. G., Kross, E., Krpan, K. M., Askren, M. K., Burson, A., Deldin, P. J., Kaplan, S., Sherdell, L., Gotlib, I. H. and Jonides, J. (2012). Interacting with nature improves cognition and affect for individuals with depression. *Journal of Affective Disorders*, 140: 300–305.

Berto, R. (2005). Exposure to restorative environments helps restore attentional capacity. *Journal of Environmental Psychology*, 25: 249–259.

Beute, F. and de Kort, Y. A. W. (2014). Salutogenic effects of the environment: Review of health protective effects of nature and daylight. *Applied Psychology: Health and Well-Being*, 6(1): 67–95, doi: 10.1111/aphw.12019.

Bird, W. (2007). *Natural Thinking: Investigating the Links between the Natural Environment, Biodiversity and Mental Health*. London: Royal Society for the Protection of Birds.

Bjørnerem, A., Straume, B., Midtby, M., Fønnebø, V., Sundsfjord, J., et al. (2004). Endogenous sex hormones in relation to age, sex, lifestyle factors, and chronic diseases in a general population: The Tromso Study. *Journal of Clinical Endocrinology and Metabolism*, 89: 6039–6047.

BMA (2011). *The Psychological and Social Needs of Patients*. London: British Medical Association.

Boden, J. M., Fergusson, D. M. and Horwood, L. J. (2008). Does adolescent self-esteem predict later life outcomes? A test of the causal role of self-esteem. *Development and Psychopathology*, 20: 319–339.

Bolton, M. (2012). *Loneliness – The State We're In*. London: Campaign to End Loneliness.

Bouchard, C., Blair, S.N. and Haskell, W. (2006). *Physical Activity and Health*, 2nd Edition. Champaign, IL; Human Kinetics.

Bowler, D., Buyung-Ali, L., Knight, T. and Pullin, A. (2010). A systematic review of the evidence for the added benefits to health of exposure to natural environments. *BMC Public Health*, 10: 456–467.

Boyle, D. and Simms, A. (2009). *The New Economics. A Bigger Picture*. London: Earthscan.

Bragg, R. (2013). *Care farming in the UK – Key Facts and Figures*. Summary report for Natural England. Colchester: University of Essex.

Bragg, R. (2014). Nature-based interventions for mental wellbeing and sustainable behaviour: the potential for green care in the UK. A thesis submitted for the degree of Doctor of Philosophy in Environmental Sciences, at the University of Essex, Colchester.

Bragg, R. and Atkins, G. (2016). *A Review of Nature-based Interventions for Mental Health Care*. Peterborough: Natural England.

Bragg, R. and Wood, C. (2013). *Measuring connection to nature in teenagers: A robust methodology for the RSPB*. Sandy: RSPB.

Bragg, R., Wood, C., Barton, J. and Pretty, J. (2012). *Let Nature Feed Your Senses: Engaging people with Nature, Food and Farming*. Stoneleigh: ESI and LEAF.

Bragg, R., Wood, C., Barton, J. and Pretty, J. (2013a). *Measuring Connection to Nature in Children Aged 8 - 12: A Robust Methodology for the RSPB*. School of Biological Sciences and Essex Sustainability Institute, University of Essex. Sandy: RSPB.

Bragg, R., Wood, C. and Barton, J. (2013b). *Ecominds: Effects on Mental Wellbeing*. London: Mind.

Bragg, R., Egginton-Metters, I., Elsey, H. and Wood, C. (2014). *Care Farming: Defining the 'Offer' in England*. Peterborough: Natural England.

Brand, S. (2010). *How Buildings Learn*. London: Penguin.

Bratman, G. N., Hamilton, J. P. and Daily, G. C. (2012). The impacts of nature experience on human cognitive function and mental health. *Annals New York Academy of Science*, 1249: 118–136.

Bratman, G. N., Hamilton, J. P., Hahn, K. S., Daily, G. C. and Gross, J. J. (2015). Nature experience reduces rumination and subgenual prefrontal cortex activation. *Proceedings of the National Academy of Science*, 112(28): 8567–8572, doi: 10.1073/pnas.1510459112.

Brendtro, L. K., Brockenleg, M., Van Bockern, S. (2005). The circle of courage and positive psychology. *Reclaiming Children and Youth*, 14: 130–136.

Brewin, W. (2015). How nature can help people with dementia feel connected. *The Guardian*, 29 October.

Bringslimark, T., Hartig, T. and Patil, G. G. (2009). The psychological benefits of indoor plants: a critical review of the experimental literature. *Journal of Environmental Psycholgy*, 29: 422–433.

British Heart Foundation (2009). *BHF Think fit! Think well! Making the case for workplace mental wellbeing*. Online at: www.bhf.org.uk/~/media/files/publications/health-at-work/z217-making-the-case-for-workplace-mental-wellbeing.pdf

Brookes, A. (2007). A critique of neo-Hahnian outdoor education theory. Part one: Challenges to the concept of 'character building'. *Journal of Adventure Education and Outdoor Learning*, 3(1): 49–62.

Brown, H. E., Gilson, N. D., Burton, N. W. and Brown, W. J. (2011). Does physical activity impact on presenteeism and other indicators of workplace well-being? *Sports Medicine*, 41: 249–262.

Brown, D. K., Barton, J. L., Pretty, J. and Gladwell, V. F. (2012). Walks4work: rationale and study design to investigate walking at lunchtime in the workplace setting. *BMC Public Health*, 12: 550.

Brown, D. K., Barton, J. L. and Gladwell, V. F. (2013). Viewing nature scenes positively affects recovery of autonomic function following acute-mental stress. *Environmental Science and Technology*, 47: 5562–5569.

Brown, D. K., Barton, J. L., Pretty, J. and Gladwell, V. F. (2014). Walks4work: Assessing the role of the natural environment in a workplace physical activity intervention. *Scandinavian Journal of Work, Environment and Health*, 40 (4): 390–399.

Brown, S. (1997). Excess mortality of schizophrenia: A meta-analysis. *British Journal of Psychiatry*, 171: 502–508.

Brownson, R. C., Boehmer, T. K. and Luke, D. A. (2005). Declining rates of physical activity in the US: what are the contributors? *Annual Review of Public Health*, 26: 421–43.

Brymer, E., Cuddihy, T. and Sharma-Brymer, V. (2010). The role of nature-based experiences in the development and maintenance of wellness. *Asia-Pacific Journal of Health, Sport and Physical Education*, 1(2): 21–27.

Brymer, E., and Davids, K. (2012). Ecological dynamics as a theoretical framework for development of sustainable behaviours towards the environment. *Environmental Education Research*, 19(1): 45–63.

Brymer, E., and Davids, K. (2014). Experiential learning as a constraint-led process: an ecological dynamics perspective. *Journal of Adventure Education & Outdoor Learning*, 14(2): 103–117.

Brymer, E., Davids, K. and Mallabon, L. (2014). Understanding the psychological health and well-being benefits of physical activity in nature: an ecological dynamics analysis. *Ecopsychology*, 6(3): 189–197.

Buck, D. and Gregory, S. (2013). *Improving the Public's Health: A Resource for Local Authorities*. London: Kings Fund.

Buckner, J. C. (1988). The development of an instrument to measure neighborhood cohesion. *American Journal of Community Psychology*, 16: 771–791.

Bull, F. C. and the Expert Working Groups (2010). *Physical Activity Guidelines in the UK: Review and Recommendations*. Loughborough: School of Sport, Exercise and Health Sciences, Loughborough University.

Burchardt, T., Le Grand, J. and Piachaud, D. (2002). Degrees of exclusion: developing a dynamic, multidimensional measure. In Hills, J., Le Grand, J. and Piachaud, D. (eds), *Understanding Social Exclusion*. New York: Oxford University Press.

Burdette, H. L. and Whittaker, R. C. (2005). Resurrecting free play in young children. *Archives of Pediatric and Adolescent Medicine*, 159: 46–50.

Byrne, J., Sipe, N. and Searle, G. (2010). Green around the gills? The challenge of density for urban greenspace planning in SEQ. *Australian Planner*, 47(3): 162–177.

Byun, K., Hyodo, K., Suwabe, K., Ochi, G., Sakari, Y., Kato, M., Dan, I. and Soya, H. (2014). Positive effect of acute mild exercise on executive function via arousal-related prefrontal activations: An FNIRS study. *Neuroimage*, 98: 336–345.

Cabinet Office and Department for Education. (2010). Positive for youth. Online at: www.gov.uk/government/publications/positive-for-youth-a-new-approach-to-cross-government-policy-for-young-people-aged-13-to-19/positive-for-youth-the-statement

Calfas, K. and Taylor, C. (1994). Effects of physical activity on psychological variables in adolescents. *Pediatric Exercise Science*, 6: 406–423.

Cama, R. (2009). *Evidence-based Healthcare Design*. Hoboken, NJ: Wiley.

Campaign to End Loneliness (2015). Campaign to End Loneliness. Online at: www.campaigntoendloneliness.org/

Cason, D.R. and Gills, H. L. (1993). A meta-analysis of adventure programming with adolescents. *Journal of Experiential Education*, 4: 25–27.

Cattell, J., Mackie, A., Prestage, Y. and Wood, M. (2013). *Results from the Offender Management Community Cohort Study* (OMCCS): *Assessment and sentence planning*. Matrix Evidence and NatCen Social Research, Ministry of Justice. Online at: www.gov.uk/government/publications/reoffending-by-offenders-on-community-orders-results-from-the-offender-management-community-cohort-study

Caulkins, M. C., White, D. D. and Russell, K. C. (2006). The role of physical exercise in wilderness therapy for troubled adolescent women. *Journal of Experiential Education*, 29: 18–37.

Centres for Disease Control and Prevention (CDC) (1996). *Physical Activity and Health. A Report of the Surgeon General*. Washington, D.C.: Centres for Disease Control and Prevention

Centres for Disease Control and Prevention (2010). *The Association between School-based Physical Activity, including Physical Education, and Academic Performance*. Atlanta, GA: U.S. Department of Health and Human Services.

Chalquist, C. (2009). A look at the ecotherapy research evidence. *Ecopsychology*, 1: 64–74.

Chan, L. (2013). Windows with a Biodiversity View. Singapore: National Biodiversity Centre. Online at: www.thenatureofcities.com/2013/04/21/windows-with-a-biodiversity-view/

Chang, C.-Y., Hammitt, W. E., Chen, P., Machnik, L. and Su, W. (2008). Psychophysiological responses and restorative values of natural environments in Taiwan. *Landscape and Urban Planning*, 85: 79–84.

Chau, J. Y., der Ploeg, H. P., van Uffelen, J. G., Wong, J., Riphagen, I., Healy, G. N., Gilson, N. D., Dunstan, D. W., Bauman, A. E., Owen, N. and Brown, W. J. (2010). Are workplace interventions to reduce sitting effective? A systematic review. *Preventive Medicine*, 51: 352–356.

Chief Medical Officer (CMO) (2013). *Our Children Deserve Better: Prevention Pays*. Chief Medical Officer's Annual Report 2012. London: UK Government.

Children and Nature Network, (2012). Health benefits to children from contact with the outdoors and nature. Children and Nature Network. Online at http://eclkc.ohs. acf.hhs.gov/hslc/tta-system/teaching/eecd/nature-based-learning/Research/health-benefits-from-outdoor.pdf

Children's Society (2012). *The Good Childhood Report 2012: A review of our children's wellbeing*. Leeds: The Children's Society.

Christiansen, C. H., Baum, C. M. and Bass-Haugen, J. (eds) (2005). *Occupational Therapy: Performance, Participation and Wellbeing*, (3rd edn). Thorofare, NJ: SLACK Incorporated.

Christie, D. E. (2013). *The Blue Sapphire of the Mind*. New York: Oxford University Press.

Cimprich, B. and Ronis, D. L. (2003). An environmental intervention to restore attention in women with newly diagnosed breast cancer. *Cancer Nursing*, 26(4): 274–292.

Clark, P., Mapes, N., Burt, J. and Preston, S. (2013). Greening dementia – a literature review of the benefits and barriers facing individuals living with dementia in accessing the natural environment and local green-space. *Natural England Commissioned Reports*, 137. Online at: http://publications.naturalengland.org.uk/file/5997922130853888

Cleland, V., Crawford, D., Baur, L. A., Hume, C., Timperio, A. and Salmon, J. (2008). A prospective examination of children's time spent outdoors, objectively measured physical activity and overweight, *International Journal of Obesity*, 32: 1685–1693.

Cobb, S. (1976). Social support as a moderator of life stress. *Psychosomatic Medicine*, 38: 300–314.

Cocker, H. (2012). The positive effects of aquarium visits on children's behaviour: A behavioural observation. *The Plymouth Student Scientist*, 5: 165–181.

Coe, D. P., Pivarnik, J. M., Womack, C. J., Reeves, M. J. and Malina, R. M. (2006). Effect of physical education and activity levels on academic achievement in children. *Medicine and Science in Sports and Exercise*, 38: 1515.

Conn, V. S., Hafdahl, A. R., Cooper, P. S., Brown, L. M. and Lusk, S. L. (2009). Meta-analysis of workplace physical activity interventions. *American Journal of Preventive Medicine*, 37: 330–339.

Connor, M. (2009). What is wilderness therapy? Princeton Online Article. Online at: www.princetonol.com/summercamps/polArticles.cfm?doc_id=1175

Cook, M. (2015). *Forests as Places of Mental Well-being for People with Dementia*. Dundee: Departments of Geography and Social Dimensions of Health Institute (SDHI), University of Dundee.

Cooper, A. R., Page, A. S., Wheeler, B. W., Griew, P., Davis, L. and Hillsdon, M. (2010). Mapping the walk to school using accelerometry combined with a Global Positioning System. *American Journal of Preventive Medicine*, 38(2): 178–183.

Cooper-Marcus, C. and Barnes, M. (1999). *Healing Gardens: Therapeutic Benefits and Design Recommendations*. New York: Wiley.

Cordell, H. K., Bergstrom, J. C. and Bowker, J. M. (2005). *The Multiple Values of Wilderness*. State College, PA: Venture Publishing, Inc.

Costanza, R., de Groot, R., Sutton, P., van der Ploeg, S., Kubiszewski, I., Farber, S. and Turner, R. K. (2014).Changes in the global value of ecosystem services. *Global Environmental Change*, 26: 152–158.

Crawford, D., Timperio, A., Giles-Corti, B., Ball, K., Hume, C., et al. (2008). Do features of public open spaces vary according to neighbourhood socio-economic status? *Health and Place*, 14: 889–893.

Creed, P. A. and Macintyre, S. R. (2001). The relative effects of deprivation of the latent and manifest benefits of employment on the wellbeing of unemployed people. *Journal of Occupational Health Psychology*, 6: 324–331.

Curasi, C. F., Price, L. L. and Arnould, E. J. (2005). How individuals' cherished possessions become families' inalienable wealth. *Journal of Consumer Research*, 31: 609–622.

Currie, C., Zanotti, C., Morgan, A., Currie, D., De Looze, M., et al. (2012). *Social Determinants of Health and Well-being among Young People. Health Behaviour in School-aged Children (HSBC) Study: International Report from the 2009/2010 Survey*. Copenhagen: World Health Organisation.

Cusson, M. and Pinsonneault, P. (1986). The decision to give up crime. In Cornish, D. B. and Clarke, R. V. (eds), *The Reasoning Criminal*. New York: Springer, Verlag.

Dadvand, P., de Nazelle, A., Figueras, F., Basagana, X., Su, J., Amoly, E., Jerrett, M., Vrijheid, M., Sunyer, J. and Nieuwenhuijsen, M. J. (2012). Green space, health inequality and pregnancy. *Environment International*, 40: 110–115.

Daffner, K. R., Mesulam, M., Scinto, L., Acar, D., Calvo, V., et al. (2000). The central role of the prefrontal cortex in directing attention to novel events. *Brain*, 123: 927–939.

Daly, H. E. and Cobb, C. (1989). *For the Common Good*. Boston, MA: Beacon Press.

Danner, D., Snowdon, D. and Friesen, W. (2001). Positive emotions in early life and longevity: Findings from the Nun Study. *Journal of Personality and Social Psychology*, 80: 804–813.

Dasgupta, P. (2010). Nature's role in sustaining economic development. *Philosophical Transactions of the Royal Society* B, 365: 5–11.

Dauchet, L., Amouyel, P. and Dallongeville, J. (2006). Fruit and vegetable consumption and risk of stroke: a meta-analysis of cohort studies. *Neurology*, 65: 1193–1197.

Davis-Berman, J. and Berman, D. S. (1994). *Wilderness Therapy: Foundations, Theories and Research*. Dubuque: IA Kendall/Hunt.

Davis-Berman, J. S. and Berman, D. S. (2008). *The Promise of Wilderness Therapy*. Boulder, CO: Association for Experiential Education.

DCLG (2012). *National planning policy framework*. London: Department for Communities and Local Government.

De Bruin, S. R., Stoop, A., Molema, C. C. M., Vaandrager, L., Hop, P. J. W. M. and Baan, C. A. (2015). Green care farms: an innovative type of adult day service to stimulate social participation of people with dementia. *Gerontology and Geriatric Medicine*, doi: 10.1177/2333721415607833.

De Vries, S., van Dillen, S. M. E., Groenewegen, P. P. and Spreeuwenberg, P. (2013). Streetscape greenery and health: Stress, social cohesion and physical activity as mediators. *Social Science and Medicine*, 94(0): 26–33, doi: 10.1016/j.socscimed.2013.06.030.

DEFRA (2011). The natural choice: Securing the value of nature. Natural Environment White Paper. London: The Stationery Office.

Department for Education (DfE) (2013). The national curriculum in England: Key Stages 1 and 2 framework document. Online at: www.gov.uk/government/uploads/system/uploads/attachment_data/file/335133/PRIMARY_national_curriculum_220714.pdf

Department for Education (DfE)(2015). *Permanent and Fixed-Period Exclusions in England: 2013–2014.* London: Office for National Statistics.

Department for Education and Early Childhood Development (2013). *The Natural Environment.* London: Department for Education and Early Childhood Development.

Department of Health (2009). *Be Active and Healthy. A Plan for Getting the Nation Moving.* London: Department for Health.

Department of Health (2011a). *Healthy Lives, Healthy People.* London: Department for Health.

Department of Health (2011b). *Start Active, Stay Active: A Report on Physical Activity from the Four Home Countries' Chief Medical Officers.* London: Department of Health.

Depledge, M. H. and Bird, W. J. (2009). The blue gym: Health and wellbeing from our coasts. *Marine Pollution Bulletin,* 58(7): 947–948.

Dietrich, A. (2006). Transient hypofrontality as a mechanism for the psychological effects of exercise. *Psychiatric Research,* 145: 79–83.

Dietrich, A. and Sparling, P. B. (2004). Endurance exercise selectively impairs prefrontal-dependent cognition. *Brain Cognition,* 55: 516–524.

Dillon, J. and Dickie, I. (2012). *Learning in the Natural Environment: Review of Social and Economic Benefits and Barriers.* Peterborough: Natural England.

Dinnie, E., Brown, K. M. and Morris, S. (2013). Community, cooperation and conflict: Negotiating the social well-being benefits of urban greenspace experiences. *Landscape and Urban Planning,* 112: 1–9.

Dishman, R. K., Sallis, J. F. and Orenstein, D. R. (1985). The determinants of physical activity and exercise. *Public Health Reports,* 100(2): 158–171.

Dow, A. (2014). Melbourne can't afford new parks, *The Age Newspaper,* 14 September.

Drake, R. and Whitley, R. (2014). Recovery and severe mental illness: description and analysis. *Canadian Journal of Psychiatry,* 59: 236–242.

Duncan, M. J., Clarke, N. D., Birch, S. L., Tallis, J., Hankey, J., Bryant, E. and Eyre, E. L. J. (2014). The effect of green exercise on blood pressure, heart rate and mood state in primary school children. *International Journal of Environmental Research and Public Health,* 11: 3678–3688.

Dusek, J. A., Sherwood, J. B., Friedman, R., Myers, P., Bethea, C. F., Levitsky, S., Hill, P. C., Jain, M. K., Kopecky, S. L., Mueller, P. S., Lam, P., Benson, H. and Hibberd, P. L. (2002). Study of the therapeutic effects of intercessory prayer (STEP): study design and research methods. *American Heart Journal,* 143(4): 577–584.

Duvall, J. (2011). Enhancing the benefits of outdoor walking with cognitive engagement strategies. *Journal of Environmental Psychology,* 31(1): 27–35.

Duvall, J. (2013). Using engagement-based strategies to alter perceptions of the walking environment. *Environment and Behavior,* 45(3): 303–322.

Dyment, J. E., Bell, A. C. (2008). Grounds for movement: Green school grounds as sites for promoting physical activity. *Health Education Research,* 23: 952–962.

Ekblom-Bak, E., Ekblom, B., Vikstrom, M., du Faire, U. and Hellenius, M. -L. (2013). The importance of non-exercise physical activity for cardiovascular health and longevity. *British Journal of Sports Medicine,* doi: 10.1136/bjsports-2012–092038.

Ekeland, E., Heian, F. and Coren, E. (2005). Can exercise improve self-esteem in children and young people? A systematic review of randomized control trials. *British Journal of Sports Medicine,* 39: 792–798.

Ekkekakis, P. and Petruzzello, S. J. (1999). Acute aerobic exercise and affect. *Sports Medicine*, 28(5): 337–347.

Ekkekakis, P., Parfitt, G. and Petruzzello, S. J. (2011). The pleasure and displeasure people feel when they exercise at different intensities. *Sports Medicine*, 41(8): 641–671.

Elings, M. (2012). *Effects of Care Farms: Scientific Research on the Benefits of Care Farms to Clients*, Wageningen: Task Force Multifunctional Agriculture, Plant Research International, Trimbos Institute and Practikon/Radboud University.

Elings, M. and Beerens, A. (2012). The added value and effects of care farms on clients with psychiatric or addiction problems. *Acta Horticulturae*, 954: 57–66.

Elsey, H., Bragg, R., Brennan, B., Murray, J., Elings, M., et al. (2014a). The impact of care farms on quality of life among different population groups: protocol for a systematic review. The Campbell Collaboration. Online at: www.campbellcollaboration.org/lib/project/321/

Elsey, H., Bragg, R., Elings, M., Cade, J. E., Brennan, C., et al. (2014b). Understanding the impacts of care farms on health and well-being of disadvantaged populations: a protocol of the Evaluating Community Orders (ECO) pilot study. *BMJ Open*, 4: e006536.

Elsey, H., Murray, J. and Bragg, R. (2015). Green fingers and clear minds: prescribing 'care farming' for mental illness. *British Journal of General Practice*, (Submitted).

Enck, P., Benedetti, F. and Schedlowski, M. (2008). New insights into the placebo and nocebo responses. *Neuron Review*, 59: 195–206.

Epstein, L. H., Raja, S., Gold, S. S., Paluch, R. A., Pak, Y. and Roemmich, J. N. (2006). Reducing sedentary behavior: The relationship between park area and the physical activity of youth. *Psychological Science*, 17: 654–659.

Erickson, K. I., Weinstein, A. M., Lopez, O. L. (2012). Physical activity, brain plasticity and Alzheimer's disease. *Archives of Medical Research*, 43: 615–621.

Esch, T. and Stefano, G. B. (2005). Love promotes health. *Neuroendocrinol Letters*, 26(3): 264–267.

Esch, T., Fricchione, G. L. and Stefano, G. B. (2003). The therapeutic use of the relaxation response in stress-related diseases. *Medical Science Monitor*, 9(2): RA23–34.

European Agency for Safety and Health at Work (2014). *Psychosocial Risks in Europe Prevalence and Strategies for Prevention*. Online at https://osha.europa.eu/en/tools-and-publications/publications/reports/psychosocial-risks-eu-prevalence-strategies-prevention

Evans, A. and Evans, S. (2015). Social healing through integrated farm therapy. Online at: www.clinks.org/sites/default/files/SHIFT%20Hereforshire%20ToC.pdf

Even, C., Schroder, C. M., Friedman, S. and Rouillon, F. (2008). Efficacy of light therapy in non-seasonal depression: a systematic review. *Journal of Affective Disorders*, 108(2): 11–23.

Ewert, A., Overholt, J., Voight, A. and Wang, C. C. (2011). Understanding the transformative aspects of the wilderness and protected lands experience upon human health. *USDA Forest Service Proceedings*, 1: 140–146.

Faber Taylor, A. and Kuo, F. E. (2011). Could exposure to everyday green spaces help treat ADHD? Evidence from children's play settings. *Applied Psychology: Health and Well-Being*, 3(3): 281–303.

Faigenbaum, A. D. and Myer, G. D. (2012). Exercise deficit disorder in youth: play now or pay later. *Current Sports Medicine Reports*, 11: 196–200.

Farrall, S. and Bowling, B. (1999). Structuration, human development and desistance from crime. *British Journal of Criminology*, 39: 253–268.

Farrall, S. and Calverley, A. (2006). *Understanding Desistance from Crime: Theoretical directions in Resettlement and Rehabilitation*. Oxford: McGraw-Hill Education, Oxford University Press.

Fawcett, N. R. and Gullone, E. (2001). Cute, cuddly and a whole lot more? A call for empirical investigation into the therapeutic benefits of human-animal interaction for children. *Behaviour Change*, 18: 124–133.

Fieldhouse, J. and Sempik, J. (2014). Occupational therapy and green care. In Banigan, K., Bryant, W. and Fieldhouse, J. (eds), *Creek's Occupational Therapy in Mental Health* (5th edn), Edinburgh: Elsevier.

Finniss, D. G., Kaptchuk, T. J., Miller, F. and Benedetti, F. (2010). Placebo effects: biological, clinical and ethical advances. *The Lancet*, 375(9715): 686–695.

Fjortoft, I. (2004). Landscape as playscape: the effects of natural environments on children's play and motor development. *Children, Youth and Environments*, 14: 23–44.

Floyd, M. F., Spengler, J. O., Maddock, J. E., Gobster, P. H. and Suau, L. J. (2008a). Environmental and social correlates of physical activity in neighborhood parks: An observational study in Tampa and Chicago. *Leisure Sciences*, 30: 360–375.

Floyd, M. F., Spengler, J. O., Maddock, J. E., Gobster, P. H. and Suau, L. J. (2008b). Park-based physical activity in diverse communities of two U.S. cities: An observational study. *American Journal of Preventive Medicine*, 34: 299–305.

Floyd, M. F., Bocarro, J. N., Smith, W. R., Baran, P. K., Moore, R. C., Cosco, N. G., Edwards, M. B., Suau, L. J. and Fang, K. (2011). Park-based physical activity among children and adolescents. *American Journal of Preventive Medicine*, 41: 258–265.

Focht, B. C. (2009). Brief walks in outdoor and laboratory environments: effects on affective responses, enjoyment, and intentions to walk for exercise. *Research Quarterly for Exercise and Sport*, 80(3): 611–620.

Forbes, D., Forbes, S. C., Blake, C. M., Thiessen, E. J. and Forbes, S. (2015). Exercise programs for people with dementia. *Cochrane Database of Systematic Reviews*, doi: 10.1002/14651858.CD006489.pub4

Foresight (2007). *Tackling Obesities: Future Choices*. London: Government Office of Science.

Foresight (2008). *Mental health – Future challenge*. London: Government Office of Science.

Forestry Commission England (2013). *Corporate plan 2013–14*, Edinburgh: Forestry Commission England.

Forestry Commission Scotland (2009). *Woods for Learning Strategy*. Edinburgh: Forestry Commission Scotland.

Fox, R. and Lloyd, W. (1938). Convalescence on the coast. *The Lancet*, 232(5992): 37–39.

Francis, J., Giles-Corti, B., Wood, L. and Knuiman, M. (2012a). Creating sense of community: The role of public space. *Journal of Environmental Psychology*, 32: 401–409.

Francis, J., Wood, L., Knuiman, M. and Giles-Corti, B. (2012b). Quality or quantity? Exploring the relationship between Public Open Space attributes and mental health in Perth, Western Australia. *Social Science and Medicine*, 74: 1570–1577.

Frankenhaeuser, M. (1975). Experimental approach to the study of catecholamines and emotion. In Levi, L. (ed.), *Emotions, Their Parameters and Measurement*. New York: Raven Press.

Friedmann, E. (1983). Animal-human bond: health and wellness. In Katcher, A. and Beck, A. (eds), *New Perspectives on Our Lives with Companion Animals*. Philadelphia, PA: University of Pennsylvania Press.

Frumkin, H. (2001). Beyond toxicity: human health and the natural environment. *American Journal of Preventive Medicine*, 20(3): 234–240.

Frumkin, H. (2004). White coats, green plants: Clinical epidemiology meets horticulture. *Acta Horticulturae*, 639: 15–26.

Frumkin, H. (ed.) (2005). *Environmental Health: From Global to Local*. San Francisco, CA: Jossey-Bass.

Frumkin, H. (2008). Nature contact and human health: building the evidence base. In Kellert, S., Heerwagen, J. and Mador, M., *Biophilic Design: The Theory, Science, and Practice of Bringing Buildings to Life*. Hoboken, NJ: Wiley.

Fuente-Fernandez, R., Ruth, T. J., Sossi, V., Calne, D. and Stoessi, A. J. (2001). Expectation and dopamine release: mechanism of the placebo effect in Parkinson's disease. *Science*, 293: 1164–1166.

Fuller, R. A., Irvine, K. N., Devine-Wright, P., Warren, P. H. and Gaston, K. J. (2007). Psychological benefits of greenspace increase with biodiversity. *Biological Letters*, 3: 390–394.

Gesler, W. M. (1993). Therapeutic landscapes: theory and a case study of Epidauros, Greece. *Environment and Planning D: Society and Space*, 11(2): 171–189.

Gidlow, C., Chochrane, T., Davey, R., Smith, G. and Fairburn, J. (2010). Relative importance of physical and social aspects of perceived neighbourhood environment for self-reported health. *Preventative Medicine*, 51: 157–163.

Giles-Corti, B., Bull, F., Knuiman, M., McCormack, G., Van Niel, K., Timperio, A., Christian, H., Foster, S., Divitini, M., Middleton, N. and Boruff, B. (2013). The influence of urban design on neighbourhood walking following residential relocation: Longitudinal results from the RESIDE study. *Social Science and Medicine*, 77: 20–30.

Gill, T. (2011). *Children and Nature*. London: Sustainable Development Commission.

Gladwell, V. F., Brown, D. K., Wood, C., Sandercock, G. R. and Barton, J. L. (2013). The great outdoors: how a green exercise environment can benefit all. *Extreme Physiology and Medicine*, 2(1): 1–7.

Glaser, R., Kiecolt-Glaser, J. K., Speicher, C. E. and Holliday, J. E. (1985). Stress, loneliness, and changes in herpes virus latency. *Journal of Behavioral Medicine*, 8(3): 1985.

Gonzalez, M. T., Hartig, T., Patil, G. G., Martinsen, E. W. and Kirkevold, M. (2009). Therapeutic horticulture in clinical depression: A prospective study. *Research and Theory for Nursing Practice*, 23: 312–328.

Goran, M. I., Nagy, T. R., Gower, B. A., Mazariegos, M., Solomons, N., Hood, V. and Johnson, R. (1998). Influence of sex, seasonality, ethnicity and geographical location on the components of total energy expenditure in young children. *American Journal of Clinical Nutrition*, 68: 675–682.

Gordon-Larsen, P., McMurray, R. G. and Popkin, B. M. (2000). Determinants of adolescent physical activity and inactivity patterns. *Pediatrics*, 105: 83–90.

Government of South Australia (2014). Healthy and strong children. Building a Stronger South Australia Policy Initiatives Paper 8, Adelaide. Online at: www.premier.sa.gov.au/strongersa

Granerud, A. and Eriksson, B. G. (2014). Mental health problems, recovery, and the impact of green care services: a qualitative, participant-focused approach. *Occupational Therapy in Mental Health*, 30: 317–336.

Green, R. (2013). Close to nature. Australian healthcare design 2005–2015: A critical review of the design and build of healthcare infrastructure in Australia. *International Academy for Design and Health, Melbourne*, 76–81.

Green Care Coalition (2015). Discussions from the Green Care Coalition Working Group. Personal communication: October 2015.

Griffiths, L. J., Parsons, T. J. and Hill, A. J. (2010). Self-esteem and quality of life in obese children and adolescents: a systematic review. *International Journal of Pediatric Obesity*, 5: 282–304.

Grinde, B. R. and Patil, G. (2009). Biophilia: Does visual contact with nature impact on health and well-being? *International Journal of Environmental Research and Public Health*, 6: 2332–2343.

Hartig, T., Book, A., Garvill, J., Olsson, T. and Garling, T. (1996). Environmental influences on psychological restoration. *Scandinavian Journal of Psychology*, 37, 378-393.

Hägerhäll, C. M. (2010). Forests, human health and well-being in light of climate change and urbanisation. *Forests and Society – Responding to Global Drivers Of Change*. Vienna, Austria: IUFRO.

Hall, J. (2004). *Phoenix House Therapeutic Conservation Programme: Underpinning Theory*. English Nature Research report 611. English Nature.

Hamilton, M. T., Healy, G. N., Dunstan, D. W., Zderic, T. W. and Owen, N. (2008). Too little exercise and too much sitting: inactivity physiology and the need for new recommendations on sedentary behavior. *Current Cardiovascular Risk Reports*, 2: 292–298.

Handley, R. (2005). Out of the bush – into the wilderness: Tension and change. A paper presented to the 6th Annual Conference on Chldren with Emotional or Behavioural Problems, Adelaide, SA.

Hans, T. A. (2000). A meta-analysis of the effects of adventure programme on locus of control. *Journal of Contemporary Psychotherapy*, 30: 33–60.

Hargrave, T. and Pfitzer, F. (2011). *Restoration Therapy*. New York: Taylor & Francis Group.

Harris, E. C. and Barraclough, B. (1998). Excess mortality of mental disorder, *British Journal of Psychiatry*, 173: 11–53.

Hart, G. D. (1965). Asclepius: god of medicine. *Canadian Medical Association*, 92: 232–236.

Hartig, T. (2008). Green space, psychological restoration, and health inequality. *The Lancet*, 372 (9650): 1614–1615.

Hartig, T. and Staats, H. (2006). The need for psychological restoration as a determinant of environmental preferences. *Journal of Environmental Psychology*, 26: 215–226.

Hartig, T., Evans, G. W., Jamner, L. D., David, D. S. and Garling, T. (2003). Tracking restoration in natural and urban settings. *Journal of Environmental Psychology*, 23: 109–123.

Hartig, T., Mitchell, R., de Vries, S. and Frumkin, H. (2014). Nature and health. *Annual Review of Public Health*, 35: 207–228.

Hassink, J., Elings, M., Zweekhorst, M., Van Den Nieuwenhuizen, N. and Smit, A. (2010). Care farms in the Netherlands: attractive empowerment-oriented and strengths-based practices in the community. *Health and Place*, 16: 423–430.

Hattie, J., Marsh, H. W., Neill, J. T. and Richards, G. E. (1997). Adventure education and outward bound out of class experiences that make a lasting difference. *Review of Educational Research*, 67: 43–87.

Hawkins, J. L., Mercer, J., Thirlaway, K. J. and Clayton, D. A. (2013). 'Doing' gardening and 'Being' at the allotment site: Exploring the benefits of allotment gardening for stress reduction and healthy aging. *Ecopsychology*, doi: 10.1089/eco.2012.0084.

Hawkley, L. C. and Cacioppo, J. T. (2007). Aging and loneliness. Downhill quickly? *Current Directions in Psychological Science*, 16(4): 187–191.

Health and Social Care Information Centre (2014). *Health Survey for England 2013*. London: Health and Social Care Information Centre.

Hellhammer, D. H., Wüst, S. and Kudielka, B. M. (2009). Salivary cortisol as a biomarker in stress research. *Psychoneuroendocrinology*, 34: 163–171.

Heritage Lottery Fund (2014). *State of UK Public Parks 2014: Renaissance to Risk?* London: Heritage Lottery Fund.

Heritage Council (n.d.). *Heritage in School*. Online at: www.heritageinschools.ie/heritage-experts/

Herzog, T. R. and Strevey, S. J. (2008). Contact with nature, sense of humor, and psychological well-being. *Environment and Behaviour*, 40: 747–776.

Herzog, T. R., Black, A. M., Fountaine, K. A. and Knotts, D. J. (1997). Reflection and attentional recovery as distinctive benefits of restorative environments. *Journal of Environmental Psychology*, 17(2): 165–170.

Herzog, T. R., Maguire, C. P. and Nebel, M. B. (2003). Assessing the restorative components of environments. *Journal of Environmental Psychology*, 23: 159–170.

Herzog, T. R., Hayes, L. J., Applin, R. C. and Weatherly, A. M. (2011a). Compatibility: An experimental demonstration. *Environment and Behavior*, 43(1): 95–105.

Herzog, T. R., Hayes, L. J., Applin, R. C. and Weatherly, A. M. (2011b). Incompatibility and mental fatigue. *Environment and Behavior*, 43(6): 827–847.

Hill Holt Wood (n.d.). Key Stage 4, Solutions 4. Online at: www.hillholtwood.com/education-learning/solutions-4/

Hine, R., Peacock, J. and Pretty, J. (2008a). Care farming in the UK: Contexts, benefits and links with therapeutic communities. *International Journal of Therapeutic Communities*, 29(3): 245–260.

Hine, R., Peacock, J. and Pretty, J. (2008b). *Evaluating the Impact of Environmental Volunteering on Behaviours and Attitudes to the Environment*. Report for BTCV Cymru April 2008.

Hine, R., Peacock, J. and Pretty, J. (2009). *Research Project: Social, Psychological and Cultural Benefits of Large Natural Habitat & Wilderness Experience: A review of current literature*. Report for the Wilderness Foundation. Online at: www.essex.ac.uk/ces/occasionalpapers/Kerry/Literature%20Review%20for%20WF.pdf

HM Government (2011). *The Natural Choice: Securing the Value of Nature*. London: HM Government.

Hoag, M. J., Massey, K. E. and Roberts, S. D. (2014). Dissecting the wilderness therapy client: Examining clinical trends, findings and patterns. *Journal of Experiential Education*, 1: 1–15.

Holt-Lunstad, J., Smith, T. B. and Layton, J. B. (2010). Social relationships and mortality risk: a meta-analytic review. *PLoS Medicine*, 7(7): e1000316.

Hossain, P., Kawar, B. and El Nahas, M. (2007). Obesity and diabetes in the developing world: A growing challenge. *New England Journal of Medicine*, 356(3): 213–215.

Hu, J., Wallace, D. C. and Tesh, A. S. (2010). Physical activity, obesity, nutritional health and quality of life in low-income hispanic adults with diabetes. *Journal of Community Health Nursing*, 27(2):70–83.

Humpel, N., Marshall, A. L., Leslie, E., Bauman, A. and Owen, N. (2004a). Changes in neighborhood walking are related to changes in perceptions of environmental attributes. *Annals of Behavioural Medicine*, 27(1): 60–67.

Humpel, N., Owen, N., Iverson, D., Leslie, E. and Bauman, A. (2004b). Perceived environment attributes, residential location, and walking for particular purposes. *American Journal of Preventive Medicine*, 26: 119–125.

Humpel, N., Owen, N., Leslie, E., Marshall, A. L., Bauman, A. E. and Sallis, J. F. (2004c). Associations of location and perceived environmental attributes with walking in neighborhoods. *American Journal of Health Promotion*, 18: 239–242.

Hyman, I. E., Boss, S. M., Wise, B. M., McKenzie, K. E. and Caggiano, J. M. (2010). Did you see the unicycling clown? Inattentional blindness while walking and talking on a cell phone. *Applied Cognitive Psychology*, 24(5): 597–607.

Iancu, S. C., Zweekhorst, M. B. M., Veltman, D. J., Van Balkom, A. and Bunders, J. F. G. (2014). Mental health recovery on care farms and day centres: a qualitative comparative study of users' perspectives. *Disability and Rehabilitation*, 36: 573–583.

Imai, K., Matsuyama, S., Miyake, S., Suga, K. and Nakachi, K. (2000). Natural cytotoxic activity of peripheral-blood lymphocytes and cancer incidence: an 11-year follow-up study of a general population. *The Lancet*, 356(9244): 1795–1799.

Imura, M., Misao, H. and Ushijima, H. (2006). The psychological effects of aromatherapy-massage in healthy postpartum mothers. *Journal of Midwifery and Women's Health*, 51(2): e21–7.

Insel, T. R. and Young, L. J. (2001). The neurobiology of attachment. *Nature Reviews Neuroscience*, 2: 129–136.

IPCC (2013). Fifth Assessment Report. *Climate Change 2013*. Gland: IPCC.

IPPR (2008). *Behind the Screen: The Hidden Life of Youth*. London: Institute for Public Policy Research.

Jackson, T. (ed.) (2006). *Earthscan Reader in Sustainable Consumption*. London: Earthscan.

Jackson, T. (2009). *Prosperity Without Growth*. London: Earthscan.

Jackson, N. J. (2014). *Lifewide Learning and Education in Universities and Colleges: Concepts and Conceptual Aids*. In Jackson, N. J. and Willis, J. (eds), *Lifewide Learing and Education in Universities and Colleges*. Online at: www.learninglives.co.uk/e-book.html

Jackson, L. E., Daniel, J., McCorkle, B., Sears, A. and Bush, K. F. (2013). Linking ecosystem services and human health: the Eco-Health Relationship Browser. *International Journal of Public Health*, doi: 10.1007/s00038–013–0482–1.

Jacobs, T. L., Epel, E. S., Lin, J., Blackburn, E. H., Wolkowitz, O. M., et al. (2011). Intensive meditation training, immune cell telomerase activity, and psychological mediators. *Psychoneuroendocrinology*, 36(5): 664–681.

Jahoda, M. (1979). The impact of employment in the 1930s and the 1970s. *Bulletin of the British Psychological Society*, 32: 309–14.

Janssen, I. and Leblanc, A. D. (2010). Systematic review of the health benefits of physical activity and fitness in school-aged children and youth. *International Journal of Behavioral Nutrition and Physical Activity*, 7: 40–56.

Janz, K., Letuchy, E., Eichenberger Gilmore, J. M., Burns, T. L., Torner, J. C., et al. (2010). Early physical activity provides sustained bone health benefits later in childhood. *Medicine and Science in Sports and Exercise*, 42: 1072–1078.

Jarrott, S. E. and Gigliotti, C. M. (2010). Comparing responses to horticultural-based and traditional activities in dementia care programs. *American Journal of Alzheimer's Disease and Other Dementias*, 25: 657–665.

Jarrott, S. E. and Gigliotti, C. M. (2011). Layers of influence: important contextual factors in directing dementia care programs. *Journal of Applied Gerontology*, 30: 113–122.

Jiang, B., Chang, C.-Y. and Sullivan, W. C. (2014). A dose of nature: Tree cover, stress reduction, and gender differences. *Landscape and Urban Planning*, 132: 26–36.

Joens-Matre, R. R., Welk, G. J., Calabro, M. A., Russell, D. W., Nicklay, E. and Hensley, L. D. (2008). Rural-urban differences in physical activity, physical fitness and overweight prevalence of children. *Journal of Rural Health*, 24: 49–54.

Johansson, M., Hartig, T. and Staats, H. (2011). Psychological benefits of walking: Moderation by company and outdoor environment. *Applied Psychology: Health and Well-Being*, 3(3): 261–280.

Joye, Y. (2007). Architectural lessons from environmental psychology: The case of biophilic architecture. *Review of General Psychology*, 11: 305–328.

Joye, Y., Pals, R., Steg, L. and Evans, B. L. (2013). New methods for assessing the fascinating nature of nature experiences. *PLoS ONE*, 8(7): e65332.

Juniper, T. (2013). *What Has Nature Ever Done for Us?* London: Profile.

Kahn, P. (1997). Developmental psychology and the biophilia hypothesis: Children's affiliation with nature. *Developmental Review*, 17: 1–61.

Kaiser Family Foundation. (2005). *The Effects of Electronic Media on Children Ages Zero to Six: A History of Research*. Menlo Park, CA: H.J. Kaiser Family Foundation.

Kaley, A. (2015). *Green Care in Agriculture: Interim Report*. Lancaster: Lancaster University.

Kam, M. C. Y. and Siu, A. M. H. (2010). Evaluation of a horticultural activity programme for persons with psychiatric illness. *Hong Kong Journal of Occupational Therapy*, 20: 80–86.

Kampman, M. T., Wilsgaard, T. and Mellgren, S. I. (2007). Outdoor activities and diet in childhood and adolescence relate to MS risk above the Arctic Circle. *Journal of Neurology*, 254: 471–7.

Kane, S. 1998 (2010). *Wisdom of the Mythtellers*. Peterborough, ON: Broadview Press.

Kaplan, R. (1993). The role of nature in the context of the workplace. *Landscape and Urban Planning*, 26: 193–201.

Kaplan, S. (1995). The restorative benefits of nature: toward an integrative framework. *Journal of Environmental Psychology*, 15: 169–182.

Kaplan, S. (2001). Meditation, restoration and the management of mental fatigue. *Environment and Behavior*, 33: 480–506.

Kaplan, R. (2007). Employees' reactions to nearby nature at their workplace: the wild and the tame. *Landscape and Urban Planning*, 82: 17–24.

Kaplan, S. and Berman, M. G. (2010). Directed attention as a common resource for executive functioning and self-regulation. *Perspectives on Psychological Science*, 5(1): 43–57.

Kaplan, R. and Kaplan, S. (1989). *The Experience of Nature: A Psychological Perspective*. New York: Cambridge University Press.

Kaplan, R., Kaplan, S. and Ryan, R. (1998). *With People in Mind: Design and Management of Everyday Nature*. Washington, D.C.: Island Press.

Kaptchuk, T. J., Kelley, J. M., Conboy, L. A., Davis, R. B., Kerr, C. E., et al. (2008). Components of placebo effect: randomised controlled trial in patients with irritable bowel syndrome. *British Medical Journal*, 336(7651): 999–1003.

Karageorghis, C. and Priest, D. L. (2008). Music in sport and exercise: An update on research and application. *The Sport Journal*, 11(3). Online at: http://thesportjournal. org/article/music-sport-and-exercise-update-research-and-application/

Katcher, A. and Wilkins, G. (1993). Dialogue with animals: its nature and culture. In Kellert, S. R. and Wilson, E. O. (eds), *The biophilia hypothesis*. Washington D.C.: Island Press, pp. 173–197.

Kaufman, J. A. (2015). A model of our contemplative nature. *Ecopsychology*, 7(3): 137–144.

Kawachi, I., Kennedy, B. P., Lochner, K. and Prothrow-Smith, D. (1997). Social capital, income inequality and mortality. *American Journal of Public Health*, 87: 1491–8.

Kellert, S. (1997). *Kinship to Mastery: Biophilia in Human Evolution and Development*. Washington, D.C.: Island Press.

Kellert, S. (2008). *Bringing Buildings to Life: Understanding and Designing the Human-nature Connection*. Washington, D.C.: Island Press.

Kellert, S. (2012). *Birthright: People and Nature in the Modern World*. New Haven, CT: Yale University Press.

Kellert, S. and Finnegan, B. (2011). *Biophilic Design: The Architecture of Life*. Online at: www.bullfrogfilms.com/catalog/biod.html

Kellert, S. and Heerwagen, J. (2008). Nature and healing: the science, theory, and promise of biophilic design. In Guenther, R. and Vittori, G. (eds), *Sustainable Healthcare Architecture*. Hoboken, NJ: Wiley.

Kellert, S. and Kahn, P. (eds) (2002). *Children and Nature*. Cambridge, MA: MIT Press.

Kellert, S. and Wilson, E. O. (1993). *The Biophilia Hypothesis*. Washington D.C.: Island Press.

Kellert, S., Heerwagen, J. and Mador, M. (2008). *Biophilic Design: The Theory, Science, and Practice of Bringing Buildings to Life*. Hoboken, NJ: Wiley.

Keniger, L. E., Gaston, K. J., Irvine, K. N. and Fuller, R. A. (2013). What are the benefits of interacting with nature? *International Journal of Environmental Research and Public Health*, 10: 913–935.

Kiecolt-Glaser, J. K., Glaser, R., Gravenstein, S., Malarkey, W. B. and Sheridan, J. (1996). Chronic stress alters the immune response to influenza virus vaccine in older adults. *Proceedings of the National Academy of Science*, 93: 3043–3047.

Kim, Y., Beets, M. W. and Welks, G. J. (2012). Everything you wanted to know about selecting the 'right' Actigraph accelerometer cut-points for youth, but…: a systematic review. *Journal of Science and Medicine in Sport*, 15(4): 311–21, doi: 10.1016/j.jsams.2011.12.001.

Kings Fund (2009). *Point of Care: Improving Patients' Experience*. London: Kings Fund.

Kingsley, J., Townsend, M. and Henderson-Wilson, C. (2009). Cultivating health and wellbeing: members' perceptions of the health benefits of a Port Melbourne community garden. *Leisure Studies*, 28(2): 207–219.

Kishi, A., Takamori, Y., Ogawa, K., Takano, S., Tomita, S., et al. (2002). Differential expression of granulysin and perforin by NK cells in cancer patients and correlation of impaired granulysin expression with progression of cancer. *Cancer Immunology and Immunotherapy*, 50: 604–614.

Knapp, M., King, D., Healey, A. and Thomas, C. (2011). Economic outcomes in adulthood and their associations with antisocial conduct, attention deficit and anxiety problems in childhood. *Journal of Mental Health Policy Economics*, 14: 137–149.

Koenig, H. G. (2000). Religion and medicine I: Historical background and reasons for separation. *International Journal of Psychiatry in Medicine*, 30(4): 385–398.

Kompier, M. A. J. and Marcelissen, F. H. G. (1990). *Handbook of Work Stress: A Systematic Approach for Organizational Practice*. Amsterdam: NIA.

KPMG – Econtech (2008). *The Cost of Physical Inactivity*. Canberra: Medibank Private.

Kuo, F. (2010). *Parks and Other Green Environments: Essential Components of a Health Human Habitat*. Washington, D.C.: National Recreation and Parks Association.

Kuo, F. E. and Sullivan, W. C. (2001). Aggression and violence in the inner city: effects of environment via mental fatigue. *Environment and Behaviour*, 33: 543–571.

Kuo, F. E. and Taylor, A. F. (2004). A potential natural treatment for attention-deficit/hyperactivity disorder: evidence from a national study. *American Journal of Public Health*, 94(9): 1580–1586.

Kuroda, K., Inoue, N., Ito, Y., Kubota, K., Sugimoto, A., Kakuda, T. and Fushiki, T. (2005). Sedative effects of the jasmine tea odor and (R)–(–)–linalool, one of its major odor components, on autonomic nerve activity and mood states. *European Journal of Applied Physiology*, 95: 107–14.

Kwan, B. M. and Bryan, A. (2010a). In-task and post-task affective response to exercise: Translating exercise intentions into behaviour. *British Journal of Health Psychology*, 15(1): 115–131.

Kwan, B. M., and Bryan, A. D. (2010b). Affective response to exercise as a component of exercise motivation: Attitudes, norms, self-efficacy, and temporal stability of intentions. *Psychology of Sport and Exercise*, 11(1): 71–79.

Labelle, V., Bosquet, L., Mekary, S. and Bherer, L. (2013). Decline in executive control during acute bouts of exercise as a function of exercise intensity and fitness level. *Brain Cognition*, 81: 10–17.

Lachowycz, K. and Jones, A. P. (2011). Greenspace and obesity: A systematic review of the evidence. *Obesity Review*, 12: 183–189.

Lachowycz, K., Jones, A. P., Page, A. S., Wheeler, B. W. and Cooper, A. R. (2012). What can global positioning systems tell us about the contribution of different types of urban greenspace to children's physical activity? *Health and Place*, 18(3): 586–594.

Lamberg, E. M. and Muratori, L. M. (2012). Cell phones change the way we walk. *Gait and Posture*, 35(4): 688–690.

Lang, T. and Rayner, G. (2012). Ecological public health: the 21st century's big idea? *British Medical Journal*, 345: e5466.

Langford, R., Bonell, C. P., Jones, H. E., Pouliou, T., Murphy, S. M., Waters, E., Komro, K. A., Gibbs, L. F., Magnus, D. and Campbell, R. (2014). The WHO health promoting school framework for improving the health and well-being of students and their academic achievement. Cochrane Database of Systematic Reviews, Issue 4. Art. No.: CD008958, doi: 10.1002/14651858.CD008958.pub2.

Larson, L. R., Whiting, J. W., Green, G. T. and Bowker, J. M. (2015). Contributions of non-urban state parks to youth physical activity: A case study in Northern Georgia. *Journal of Park and Recreation Administration*, 33: 2–36.

Laumann, K., Garling, T. and Stormark, K. M. (2003). Selective attention and heart rate responses to natural and urban environments. *Journal of Environmental Psychology*, 23: 125–134.

Lawrence, A., Ambrose-Oji, B. and O'Brien, L. (2014). *FES Health Check of Community Engagement*. Farnham: Report to Forestry Commission Scotland.

Layard, R. (2006). *Happiness*. London: Penguin.

Leather, P., Pyrgas, M., Beale, D. and Lawrence, C. (1998). Windows in the workplace – sunlight, view, and occupational stress. *Environment and Behavior*, 30: 739–762.

Leff, H. L. (1984). *Playful Perception: Choosing how to Experience your World*. Burlington, VT: Waterfront Books.

Lee, M. J. (2010). Effects of various horticultural activities on the autonomic nervous system and cortisol response of mentally challenged adults. *HortTechnology*, 20: 971–976.

Lee, J., Park, B. J., Tsunetsugu, Y., Ohira, T., Kagawa, T. and Miyazaki, Y. (2011). Effect of forest bathing on physiological and psychological responses in young Japanese male subjects. *Public Health*, 125: 93–100.

Lee, J., Li, Q., Tyrväinen, L., Tsunetsugu, Y., Park, B.-J., et al. (2012). Nature therapy and preventive medicine. *Public Health – Social and Behavioral Health*, 16: 325–350.

Lee, J., Tsunetsugu, Y., Takayama, N., Park, B.-J., Li, Q., et al. (2014). Influence of forest therapy on cardiovascular relaxation in young adults. *Evidence Based Complementary and Alternative Medicine*, doi: 10.1155/2014/834360

Lee, K. E., Williams, K. J. H., Sargent, L. D., Williams, N. S. G. and Johnson, K. A. (2015). 40-second green roof views sustain attention: The role of micro-breaks in attention restoration. *Journal of Environmental Psychology*, 42: 182–189.

Lenček, L. and Bosker, G. (1998). *The Beach: The History of Paradise on Earth*. New York: Viking.

Lester, S. and Maudsley, M. (2007). Play Naturally: A Review of Children's Natural Play. Play England and National Children's Bureau. Online at: www.playengland.org.uk/resource/play-naturally-a-review-of-childrens-natural-play

Li, Q. (2000). Effect of forest bathing trips on human immune function. *Environmental Health Preventive Medicine*, 15: 9–17.

Li, Q. (ed.) (2012). *Forest Medicine*. New York: Nova Science Publishers Inc.

Li, Q. and Kawada, T. (2011a). Effect of forest environments on human natural killer (NK) activity. *International Journal of Immunopathology and Pharmacology*, 24(S1): 39–44.

Li, Q. and Kawada, T. (2011b). Effect of forest therapy on the human psycho-neuro-endocrino-immune network. *Nihon Eiseigaku Zasshi*, 66: 645–50. [in Japanese].

Li, Q. and Kawada, T. (2014). The possibility of clinical applications of forest medicine. *Nihon Eiseigaku Zasshi*, 69: 117–21. [in Japanese].

Li, D. and Sullivan, W. C. (2016). Views to school landscapes and student performance: Pathways through attention restoration and stress recovery. *Landscape and Urban Planning*. Online at: https://aslathedirt.files.wordpress.com/2016/01/li-sullivan.pdf

Li, Q., Liang, Z., Nakadai, A. and Kawada, T. (2005). Effect of electric foot shock and psychological stress on activities of murine splenic natural killer and lymphokine-activated killer cells, cytotoxic T lymphocytes, natural killer receptors and mRNA transcripts for granzymes and perforin. *Stress*, 8: 107–116.

Li, Q., Nakadai, A., Matsushima, H., Miyazaki, Y. and Krensky, A. M., et al. (2006). Phytoncides (wood essential oils) induce human natural killer cell activity. *Immunopharmacology Immunotoxicology*, 28: 319–333.

Li, Q., Morimoto, K., Nakadai, A., Inagaki, H. and Katsumata, M., et al. (2007). Forest bathing enhances human natural killer activity and expression of anti-cancer proteins. *International Journal of Immunopathology and Pharmacology*, 20(S2): 3–8.

Li, Q., Morimoto, K., Kobayashi, M., Inagaki, H. Katsumata, M. et al. (2008a). Visiting a forest, but not a city, increases human natural killer activity and expression of anti-cancer proteins. *International Journal of Immunopathology and Pharmacology*, 21: 117–128.

Li, Q., Morimoto, K., Kobayashi, M., Inagaki, H. Katsumata, M. et al. (2008b). A forest bathing trip increases human natural killer activity and expression of anti-cancer proteins in female subjects. *Journal of Biological Regulators and Homeostatic Agents*, 22: 45-55. Online at: www.natureandforesttherapy.org/uploads/8/1/4/4/8144400/_forest_bathing_tripfemale_subjects_2008.pdf

Li, Q., Kobayashi, M. and Kawada, T. (2008c). Relationships between percentage of forest coverage and standardized mortality ratios (SMR) of cancers in all prefectures in Japan. *The Open Public Health Journal*, 1: 1–7.

Li, Q., Kobayashi, M., Wakayama, Y., Inagaki, H., Katsumata, M. et al. (2009). Effect of phytoncide from trees on human natural killer function. *International Journal Immunopathology and Pharmacology*, 22: 951–959.

Li, Q., Kobayashi, M., Inagaki, H., Hirata, Y., Li, Y.-J. et al. (2010). A day trip to a forest park increases human natural killer activity and the expression of anti-cancer proteins in male subjects. *Journal of Biology and Regulatory Homeostatic Agents*, 24: 157–165.

Li, Q., Otsuka, T., Kobayashi, M., Wakayama, Y., Inagaki, H., et al. (2011). Acute effects of walking in forest environments on cardiovascular and metabolic parameters. *European Journal of Applied Physiology*, 111(11): 2845–2853.

Lim, J., Amado, A., Sheehan, L. and Van Emmerik, R. (2015). Dual task interference during walking: The effects of texting on situational awareness and gait stability, *Gait and Posture*, doi: 10.1016/j.gaitpost.2015.07.060

Lin, B. B., Fuller, R. A., Bush, R., Gaston, K. J. and Shanahan, D. F. (2014a). Opportunity or orientation? Who uses urban parks and why. *PLoS ONE*, 9(1): e87422, doi: 10.1371/journal.pone.0087422

Lin, Y. H., Tsai, C. C., Sullivan, W. C., Chang, P. J. and Chang, C. Y. (2014a). Does awareness effect the restorative function and perception of street trees? *Frontiers in Psychology*, 5: 906.

Lincolnshire County Council. (n.d.). *Solutions 4: Vocational and educational training.* Online at: www.lincolnshire.gov.uk/solutions-4/84876.article

Liu, J., Bennett, K. J., Harun, N. and Probst, J. C. (2008). Urban-rural differences in overweight status and physical inactivity among US children aged 10–17 years. *The Journal of Rural Health*, 24: 407–415.

Liu, J., Jones, S. J., Probst, J. C., Merchant, A. T. and Cavicchia, P. (2012). Diet, physical activity and sedentary behaviors as risk factors for childhood obesity: An urban and rural comparison. *Journal of Childhood Obesity*, 8: 440–448.

Lottrup, L., Stigsdotter, U. K., Meilby, H. and Corazon, S. S. (2012). Associations between use, activities and characteristics of the outdoor environment at workplaces. *Urban Forestry and Urban Greening*, 11(2): 159–168.

Lottrup, L., Grahn, P. and Stigsdotter, U. K. (2013). Workplace greenery and perceived level of stress: Benefits of access to a green outdoor environment at the workplace. *Landscape and Urban Planning*, 110: 5–11.

Loucaides, C. A., Chedzoy, S. and Bennett, N. (2004). Differences in physical activity levels between urban and rural school children in Cyprus. *Health Education Research*, 19: 138–147.

Loukaitou-Sideris, A. and Sideris, A. (2010). What brings children to the park? Analysis and measurement of the variables affecting children's use of parks. *Journal of the American Planning Association*, 76: 89–107.

Louv, R. (2005). *Last Child in the Woods: Saving Our Children from Nature-Deficit Disorder.* Chapel Hill, NC: Algonquin Books.

Louv, R. (2008). *Last Child in the Woods: Saving Our Children from Nature-Deficit Disorder* (2nd edn). Chapel Hill, NC: Algonquin Books.

Louv, R. (2012). *The Nature Principle: Reconnecting with Life in a Virtual Age.* Chapel Hill, NC: Algonquin Press.

Lovasi, G. S., Quinn, J. W., Neckerman, K. M., Perzanowski, M. S. and Rundle, A. (2008). Children living in areas with more street trees have lower asthma prevalence. *Journal of Epidemiology of Community Health*, 62: 647–649.

Lovell, R. and Roe, J. (2009). Physical and mental health benefits of participation in forest school. *Countryside Recreation*, 17(1): 20–23.

Lutz, A., Brefczynski-Lewis, J., Johnstone, T. and Davidson, R. J. (2008). Regulation of the neural circuitry of emotion by compassion meditation: effects of meditative expertise. *PLoS ONE*, 3(3): e1897.

Maas, J., Verheij, R. A., Groenewegen, P. P., De Vries, S. and Spreeuwenberg, P. (2006). Green space, urbanity and health: How strong is the relation? *Journal of Epidemiology and Community Health*, 60: 587–592.

Maas, J., van Dillen, S. M. J., Verheij, R. A. and Groenewegen, P. P. (2009a). Social contacts as a possible mechanism behind the relation between green space and health. *Health and Place*, 15: 586–595.

Maas, J., Verheij, R. A., de Vries, S., Spreeuwenberg, P., Schellevis, F. G. and Groenewegen, P. P. (2009b). Morbidity is related to a green living environment. *Journal of Epidemiology and Community Health*, 63: 967–973.

McCloughlan, P., Batt, W. H., Costine, M. and Scully, D. (2011). *Second European Quality of Life Survey. Participation in Volunteering and Unpaid Work.* Dublin: European Foundation for the Improvement of Living and Working Conditions.

McEwen, B. S. (1998). Stress, adaptation, and disease: Allostasis and allostatic load. *Annals of the New York Academy of Sciences*, 840: 33–44.

McEwen, B. S. and Seeman, T. (1999). Protective and damaging effects of mediators of stress. Elaborating and testing the concepts of allostasis and allostatic load. *Annals of the New York Academy of Sciences*, 896: 30–47.

McEwen, B. S. and Stellar, E. (1993). Stress and the individual. Mechanisms leading to disease. *Archives of International Medicine*, 153: 2093–2101.

Mackay, H. (2007). *Advance Australia … where? : how we've changed, why we've changed, and what will happen next?* Sydney: Hachette Livre.

McNair, D. M., Lorr, M. and Droppleman, L. F. (1971). *Manual: Profile of mood states.* San Diego, CA: Educational and Industrial Testing Service.

McNeill, F. and Weaver, B. (2010). *Changing Lives? Desistance Research and Offender Management.* Glasgow: Scottish Centre for Crime and Justice Research and Glasgow School of Social Work.

Mahdjoubi, L. and Spencer, B. (2015). Healthy play for all ages in public open spaces. In *Handbook of Planning for Health and Wellbeing.* Oxon: Routledge.

Mahidin, A. M. M. and Maulan, S. (2012). Understanding Children Preferences of Natural Environment as a Start for Environmental Sustainability. *Procedia-Social and Behavioral Sciences*, 38: 324–333.

Maller, C., Townsend, M., Brown, P. and St Leger, L. (2002). *Healthy Parks, Healthy People: The Health Benefits of Contact with Nature in a Park Context.* Melbourne: Deakin University.

Maller, C., Townsend, M., St Leger, L., Henderson-Wilson, C., Pryor, A., Prosser, L. and Moore, M. (2008). *Healthy Parks, Healthy People: The Health Benefits of Contact with Nature in a Park Context*, (2nd edn). Melbourne: Deakin University and Parks Victoria.

Malone, K. and Tranter, P. (2003). Children's environmental learning and the use, design and management of schoolgrounds. *Children, Youth and Environments*, 13(2): 87–137.

Manura, S. (2001). *Making Good: How Ex-convicts Reform and Rebuild their Lives.* Washington D.C.: APA Books.

Mao, G. X., Cao, Y. B., Lan, X. G., He, Z. H., Chen, Z. M. et al. (2012a). Therapeutic effect of forest bathing on human hypertension in the elderly. *Journal of Cardiology*, 60: 495–502.

Mao, G. X., Lan, X. G., Cao, Y. B., Chen, Z. M., He, Z. H. et al. (2012b). Effects of short-term forest bathing on human health in a broad-leaved evergreen forest in Zhejiang Province, China. *Biomedical and Environmental Sciences*, 2012(25): 317–324.

Mapes, N. (2011). *Wandering in the Woods – a Visit Woods pilot project.* Colchester: Dementia Adventure. Online at: www.dementiaadventure.co.uk/uploads/wandering-in-the-woods-a-visit-woods-pilot-project-v-1-0.pdf

Mapes, N. (2012). *Fit as a Fiddle.* Dementia Legacy resource pack (with Age UK London).

Mapes, N. (2012). Living with dementia through the changing seasons. In Marshall, M. and Gilliard, J. (eds), *Fresh Air on my Face: Enabling people living with dementia to reconnect with nature.* London: Jessica Kingsley Publishers.

Mapes, N. (2014). Getting out and about in the British countryside: Dementia adventure. In Marshall, M. and Gilliard, J. (eds), *Creating Culturally Appropriate Outside Spaces and Experiences for People Living with Dementia*. London: Jessica Kingsley Publishers.

Mapes, N. and Hine, R. (2011). *Living with dementia and connecting with nature – exploring the benefits of green exercise with people living with dementia*. Colchester: Dementia Adventure. Online at: www.dementiaadventure.co.uk/uploads/green-exercise-and-dementia-neil-mapes-february-2011.pdf

Mapes, N. and Vale, T. (2012). *Wood if we could – Enabling groups to benefit from visiting woods*. Colchester: Dementia Adventure. Online at: http://www.dementiaadventure.co.uk/uploads/Wood%20if%20we%20could%20(1).pdf

Marcus, C. M. and Sachs, N. A. (2014). *Therapeutic Landscapes: an Evidence-based Approach to Designing Healing Gardens and Restorative Outdoor Spaces*. Hoboken, NJ: Wiley.

Marmot, M. (2010). Fair society, healthy lives: A strategic review of health inequalities in England post-2010. *Institute of Health Equity*. Online at: www.instituteofhealthequity.org/projects/fair-society-healthy-lives-the-marmot-review/fair-society-healthy-lives-full-report

Marmot, M. and Brunner, E. (2004). Cohort profile: the Whitehall II study. *International Journal of Epidemiology*, 34: 251–256.

Marmot Review (2008). *Fair society, healthy lives*. London: UCL.

Marselle, M. R., Irvine, K. N. and Warber, S. L. (2013). Walking for well-being: Are group walks in certain types of natural environments better for well-being than group walks in urban environments? *International Journal of Environmental Research and Public Health*, 10: 5603–5628.

Marshall, D. and Wakeham, C. (2015). *SHIFT Care Farm: Evaluation report for one cohort of offenders under the SHIFT Pathways approach for the use of a care farm for the management of offenders*. Online at: www.bulmerfoundation.org.uk/download/shift-evaluation

Matsuoka, R. H. (2010). Student performance and high school landscapes: Examining the links. *Landscape and Urban Planning*, 97: 273–282.

Mayer, F. S. and Frantz, C.M. (2004). The connectedness to nature scale: A measure of individuals' feeling in community with nature. *Journal of Environmental Psychology*, 24: 503–515.

Mayer, F. S., Frantz, C. M., Bruehlman-Senecal, E. and Dolliver, K. (2008). Why is nature beneficial? The role of connectedness to nature. *Environment and Behavior*, 41(5): 607–643.

Maynard, T. and Waters, J. (eds) (2014). *Exploring Outdoor Play in the Early Years*. Maidenhead: Open University Press.

MEA (Millennium Ecosystem Assessment) (2005). *Ecosystems and Human Well-Being*. Washington D.C.: Island Press.

Mellor, D., Hayashi, Y., Stokes, M., Firth, L., Lake, L., et al. (2009). Volunteering and its relationship with personal and neighborhood well-being. *Nonprofit and Voluntary Sector Quarterly*, 38(1): 144–159.

Mena-Martín, F. J., Martín-Escudero, J. C., Simal-Blanco, F., Carretero-Ares, J. L., Arzúa-Mouronte, D., Castrodeza Sanz, J. J. and Hortega Study Investigators. (2006). Influence of sympahetic activity on blood pressure and vascular damage evaluated by means of urinary albumin excretion. *Journal of Clinical Hypertension* (Greenwich), 2006(8): 619–624.

Mercer, N., Wegerif, R. and Dawes, L. (1999). Children's talk and the development of reasoning in the classroom. *British Educational Research Journal*, 25(1): 95–111.

Merchant, S., Quinn, J. and Waite, S. (2013). Final report for Exmoor National Park Authority and Institute of Health and Community. *Social and Economic Aspirations of Young People on and around Exmoor National Park*. Plymouth: Plymouth University.

Millard, P. H. and Smith, C. S. (1981). Personal belonging - a positive effect? *Gerontologist*, 21: 85–90.

Miller, G. (2011). Why loneliness is hazardous to your health. *Science*, 331: 138–140.

Miller, E. K. and Cohen, J. D. (2001). An integrative theory of prefrontal cortex function. *Annual Review of Neuroscience*, 24: 167–202.

Ministry of Justice (2013a). *Transforming Rehabilitation: A strategy for reform*. Online at: https://consult.justice.gov.uk/digital-communications/transforming-rehabilitation/results/transforming-rehabilitation-response.pdf

Ministry of Justice (2013b). *Transforming Rehabilitation: a summary of the evidence on reducing re-offending*. Online at: www.gov.uk/government/publications/transforming-rehabilitation-a-summary-of-evidence-on-reducing-reoffending

Ministry of Justice (2015). *Youth Justice Statistics 2013/2014, England and Wales*. Online at: www.gov.uk/government/uploads/system/uploads/attachment_data/file/399379/youth-justice-annual-stats-13-14.pdf

Misra, S. and Stokols, D. (2012). Psychological and Health Outcomes of Perceived Information Overload. *Environment and Behavior*, 44(6): 737–759.

Mitchell, R. (2013). Is physical activity in natural environments better for mental health than physical activity in other environments? *Sports Science and Medicine*, 91: 130–134.

Mitchell, R. and Popham, F. (2008). Effect of exposure to natural environment on health inequalities: an observational population study. *The Lancet*, 372(9650): 1655–1660.

Mizuno-Matsumoto, Y., Kobashi, S., Hata, Y., Ishikawa, O. and Asano, F. (2008). Horticultural therapy has beneficial effects on brain functions in cerebrovascular diseases. *International Journal of Intelligent Computing in Medical Sciences and Image Processing*, 2(3): 169–182.

Moksnes, U. K., Moljord, I. E. O., Espnes, G. A. and Byrne, D. G. (2010). The association between stress and emotional states in adolescents: The role of gender and self-esteem. *Personality and Individual Differences*, 49: 430–435.

Molnar, B. E., Gortmaker, S. L., Bull, F. C. and Buka, S. L. (2003). Unsafe to play? Neighborhood disorder and lack of safety predict reduced physical activity among urban children and adolescents. *American Journal of Health Promotion*, 18: 378–387.

Mooneyham, B. W. and Schooler, J. W. (2013). The costs and benefits of mind-wandering: a review. *Canadian Journal of Experimental Psychology*, 67(1): 11–18.

Moore, E. O. (1982). A prison environment's effect on health care service demands. *Journal of Environmental Systems*, 11(1): 17–34.

Moore, H. J., Nixon, C. A., Lake, A. A., Douthwaite, W., O'Malley, C. L., et al. (2014). The environment can explain differences in adolescents' daily physical activity levels living in a deprived urban area: cross-sectional study using accelerometry, GPS and focus groups. *Journal of Physical Activity and Health*, 11(8): 1517–1524, doi: 10.1123/jpah.2012-0420

Morita, E., Fukuda, S., Nagano, J., Hamajima, N., Yamamoto, H., et al. (2007). Psychological effects of forest environments on healthy adults: Shinrin-yoku (forest-air bathing, walking) as a possible method of stress reduction. *Public Health*, 121: 54–63.

Morris, J., Marzano, M., Dandy, N. and O'Brien, L. (2012). *Forestry, Sustainable Behaviours and Behaviour Change. Lessons learnt from interventions and evaluations*. Farnham: Forest Research.

Morse, N. C. and Weiss, R. S. (1955). The function and meaning of work and the job, *American Sociological Review*, 20: 191–198.

Moss, S. (2012). *Natural Childhood*. The National Trust. Online at: www.nationaltrust. org.uk/documents/read-our-natural-childhood-report.pdf

Muir, J. (1901). *Our National Parks*. Houghton, Mifflin and Company, Cambridge, MA: The Riverside Press.

Mujahid, M. S., Diez Roux, A. V., Morenoff, J. D., Raghunathan, T. E., Cooper, R. S., et al. (2008). Neighborhood characteristics and hypertension. *Epidemiology*, 19(4):590–598.

Munoz, S. A. (2009). *Children in the outdoors A literature review*. Edinburgh: Sustainable Development Research Centre.

Murray, R. and O'Brien, E. (2005). *Such Enthusiasm – a joy to see: an evaluation of Forest School in England*. Report for the Forestry Commission.

Mygind, E. (2013). *6.78 millioner bevilget til udeskole forskning [6.78 million awarded to research in udeskole]*. Health and Social Care Information Centre. Online at: http:// nexs.ku.dk/nyheder/2013-nyheder/1trygfonden-udeskole/

Natcen (2013). *Evaluation of National Citizen Service: Findings from the evaluation of the 2012 summer and autumn NCS programmes*. London: Natcen.

National Child Measurement Programme. (2013). *National Child Measurement Programme - England, 2012–13 school year*, [NS] Health and Social Care Information Centre. Online at: www.hscic.gov.uk/catalogue/PUB13115

National Environmental Education and Training Foundation (NEETF) (2000). *Environment-based Education - creating high performance schools and students*. Online at: www.promiseofplace.org/assets/files/research/NEETF8400.pdf

National Institute for Health and Care Excellence (2008). *Physical activity and the environment*. London: NICE. Online at: www.nice.org.uk/guidance/ph8

National Institute for Health and Care Excellence (2009). *Promoting mental wellbeing through productive and healthy working conditions: public health guidance 22 for employers*. In NICE public health guidance 22. London: NICE. Online at: www.nice.org.uk/ guidance/ph22/resources/mental-wellbeing-at-work-1996233648325

Natural England (2009a). *Childhood and nature: A survey on changing relationships with nature across generations*. Cambridgeshire: Natural England.

Natural England (2009b). *Our Natural Health Service The role of the natural environment in maintaining healthy lives*. Peterborough: Natural England.

Natural England (2011). *NECR084 - Monitor of Engagement with the Natural Environment: The National Survey on People and the Natural Environment - Technical Report (2010–11 survey)*. Online at: http://publications.naturalengland.org.uk/publication/46012

Natural England (2012). *Monitor of Engagement with the Natural Environment survey 2009–2012. Analysis of data related to visits with children*. Peterborough: Natural England.

Natural England (2013). *Monitor of Engagement with the Natural Environment: The national survey on people and the natural environment*. Annual Report from the 2012–13 survey. Peterborough: Natural England.

Natural England (2015). *Monitor of Engagement with the Natural Environment*. Cambridgeshire: Natural England.

NEA (National Ecosystem Assessment) (2011) The UK National Ecosystem Assessment: technical report. UNEPWCMC, Cambridge.

NEF (New Economics Foundation) (2013). *Happy Planet Index*. Online at: www. happyplanetindex.org

Neill, J. T. (2003). Reviewing and benchmarking adventure therapy outcomes: Applications of meta-analysis. *Journal of Experiential Education*, 25(3): 316–321.

Ng, S. W. and Popkin, B. (2012). Time use and physical activity: a shift away from movement across the globe. *Obesity Reviews*, 13(8): 659–680.

NHS (2015). *NHS Reference Costs 2014*. London: Department of Health.

NICE (2009). *Promoting Physical Activity for Children and Young People*. London: NICE.

Nisbet, E., Zelenski, J. and Murphy, S. (2009). The Nature Relatedness Scale: Linking Individuals' Connection with Nature to Environmental Concern and Behavior. *Environment and Behavior*, 41(5): 715–740.

Norton, C. L. and Watt, T. T. (2014). Exploring the impact of a wilderness-based positive youth development program for urban youth. *Journal of Experiential Education*, 37: 335–350.

Nyklíček, I. and Kuijpers, K. F. (2008). Effects of mindfulness-based stress reduction intervention on psychological well-being and quality of life: is increased mindfulness indeed the mechanism? *Annals of Behaviour Medicine*, 35: 331–340.

O'Brien, E. (2005a). Tackling youth disaffection through woodland vocational training. *Quarterly Journal of Forestry*, 99: 125–130.

O'Brien, E. (2005b). Bringing together ideas of social enterprise, education and community woodland: the hill holt wood approach. *Scottish Forestry*, 59: 7–14.

O'Brien, L. (2009). Learning outdoors: The Forest School approach. *Education 3–13*, 37(1): 46–60.

O'Brien, L. (2014). *Innovative NHS Greenspace. Briefing Note*. Forest Research and Forestry Commission Scotland.

O'Brien, L. and Morris, J. (2013). Well-being for all? The social distribution of benefits gained from woodlands and forests in Britain. *Local Environment*, 19(4): 356–383.

O'Brien, E. and Murray, R. (2007). Forest School and its impacts on young children: case studies in Britain. *Urban Forestry and Urban Greening*, 6: 249–265.

O'Brien, L., Townsend, M. and Ebden, M. (2010) 'Doing something positive': Volunteer's experiences of the well-being benefits derived from practical conservation activities in nature. *Voluntas: International Journal of Voluntary and Non-profit organisations*, 21: 525–545.

O'Brien, L., Burls, A., Townsend, M. and Ebden, M. (2011). Volunteering with nature as a way of enabling people to re-integrate into society. *Perspectives in Public Health*, 131: 71–81.

O'Brien, L. Morris, J. and Stewart, A. (2014). Engaging with peri-urban woodlands in England: the contribution to people's health and wellbeing and implications for future management. *International Journal of Environmental Research and Public Health*, 11: 6171–6192.

O'Connor, J. and Brown, A. (2013). A qualitative study of 'fear' as a regulator of children's independent physical activity in the suburbs. *Health and Place*, 24: 157–164.

O'Donnell, G., Deaton, A., Durand, M., Halpern, D. and Layard, R. (2014). *Wellbeing and Policy*. London: Legatum Institute.

O'Neill, D. W., Dietz, R. and Jones, N. (eds) (2010). *Enough is Enough. Ideas for a Sustainable Economy in a World of Finite Resources*. Report of the Steady State Economy Conference. Leeds: Centre for Advancement of Steady State Economy and Economic Justice for All.

O'Reilly, P. O. and Handforth, J. R. (1955). Occupational therapy with 'refractory' patients, *American Journal of Psychiatry*, 111: 763–766.

Oberhelman, S. M. (2013). *Anatomical votive reliefs as evidence for specialization at healing sanctuaries in the ancient Mediterranean world.* ATINER'S Conference Paper Series, No: HSC2013–0429, Athens.

OFCOM (2011). Teenagers would rather lose TV than internet or mobile – survey. *The Guardian.* 25 October. Online at: www.guardian.co.uk/technology/2011/oct/25/teenagers-lose-tv-internet-mobile

Ofsted (2008). *Learning Outside the Classroom: how far should you go?.* Online at: www.ofsted.gov.uk/resources/learning-outside-classroom

Öhman, A. (1986). Face the beast and fear the face: animal and social fears as prototypes for evolutionary analyses of emotion. *Psychophysiology.* 23(2): 123–145.

Ohtsuka, Y., Yabunaka, N. and Takayama, S. (1998). Shinrin-yoku (forest-air bathing and walking) effectively decreases blood glucose levels in diabetic patients. *International Journal of Biometeorology,* 41: 125–127.

ONS (2013). *Measuring National Well-being - What matters most to Personal Well-being?* London: Office for National Statistics.

Orr, D. W. (2006). *Design on the Edge.* Cambridge, MA: MIT Press.

Orth, U., Robins, R. and Meier, L. L. (2009). Disentangling the effects of low self-esteem and stressful life events on depression: Findings from three longitudinal studies. *Journal of Personality and Social Psychology,* 97: 307–321.

Osborne, R. H., Elsworth, G. R. and Whitfield, K. (2007). The Health Education Impact Questionnaire (heiQ): an outcomes and evaluation measure for patient education and self-management interventions for people with chronic conditions, *Patient Education and Counselling,* 66(2): 192–201.

Ostrom, E. (1990). *Governing the Commons: The Evolution of Institutions for Collective Action.* Cambridge: Cambridge University Press.

Ottosson, J. and Grahn, P. (2005). A comparison of leisure time spent in a garden with leisure time spent indoors: On measures of restoration in residents in geriatric care. *Landscape Research,* 30: 23–55.

Ozuner, H. (2011). Cultural differences in attitudes towards urban parks and green spaces. *Landscape Research,* 36: 599–620.

Paquette, L., Brassard, A., Guerin, A., Fortin-Chevalier, J. and Tanquay-Beaudoin, J. (2014). Effects of a developmental adventure on the self-esteem of college students. *Journal of Experiential Education,* 37: 216–231.

Park, B.-J., Tsunetsugu, Y., Kasetani, T., Hirano, H., Kagawa, T., et al. (2007). Physiological effects of Shinrin-yoku (taking in the atmosphere of the forest)--using salivary cortisol and cerebral activity as indicators. *Journal of Physiological Anthropology,* 26: 123–128.

Park, B.-J., Tsunetsugu, Y., Ishii, H., Furuhashi, S., Hirano, H., et al. (2008). Physiological effects of Shinrin-yoku (taking in the atmosphere of the forest) in a mixed forest in Shinano Town, Japan. *Scandinavian Journal of Forest Research,* 23: 278–283.

Park, B.-J., Tsunetsugu, Y., Kasetani, T., Kagawa, T. and Miyazaki, Y. (2010). The physiological effects of Shinrin-yoku (taking in the forest atmosphere or forest bathing): evidence from field experiments in 24 forests across Japan. *Environmental Health and Preventative Medicine;* 15(1): 18–26.

Parkinson, S., Lowe, C. and Vecsey, T. (2011). The therapeutic benefits of horticulture in a mental health service. *The British Journal of Occupational Therapy,* 74: 525–534.

Parr, H. (2007). Mental health, nature work, and social inclusion. *Environment and Planning D: Society and Space,* 25: 537–561.

Passy, R. and Waite, S. (2011). School Gardens and Forest Schools. In Waite, S. (ed.), *Children Learning outside the Classroom from Birth to Eleven*. London: Sage.

Passy, R., Morris, M. and Reed, F. (2010). *Impact of School Gardening on Learning*. Royal Horticultural Society. Online at: www.nfer.ac.uk/publications/RHS01/RHS01_home. cfm

Patel, V., Flisher, A. J., Hetrick, S. and McGorry, P. (2007). Mental health of young people: a global public-health challenge. *The Lancet*, 369(9569): 1302–1313.

Paxton, P. and McAvoy, L. (2000). Social psychological benefits of a wilderness adventure programme. *USDA Forest Proceedings*, 3: 202–206.

Peacock, J., Hine, R. and Pretty, J. (2007). *Got the Blues, then Find some Greenspace: The Mental Health Benefits of Green Exercise Activities and Green Care*. Colchester: University of Essex.

Peacock, J., Hine, R. and Pretty, J. (2008). The TurnAround 2007 Project. Report for the Wilderness Foundation, University of Essex.

Pearce, M., Page, A. S., Griffin, T. P. and Cooper, A. R., (2014). Who children spend time with after school: associations with objectively recorded indoor and outdoor physical activity. *International Journal of Behavioral Nutrition and Physical Activity*, 11: 45, doi: 10.1186/1479-5868-11-45.

Pedersen, I., Nordaunet, T., Martinsen, E. W., Berget, B. and Braastad, B. O. (2011). Farm animal-assisted intervention: relationship between work and contact with farm animals and change in depression, anxiety, and self-efficacy among persons with clinical depression. *Issues in mental health nursing*, 32: 493–500.

Pedersen, I., Ihlebæk, C. and Kirkevold, M. (2012a). Important elements in farm animal-assisted interventions for persons with clinical depression: a qualitative interview study. *Disability and Rehabilitation*, 34(18): 1526–1534.

Pedersen, I., Martinsen, E. W., Berget, B. and Braastad, B. O. (2012b). Farm animal-assisted intervention for people with clinical depression: A randomized controlled trial. *Anthrozoos*, 25: 149–160.

Pedretti-Burls, A. (2007). Ecotherapy: a therapeutic and educative model. *Journal of Mediterranean Ecology*, 8: 19–25.

Pedretti-Burls, A. (2008). Seeking Nature: A Contemporary Therapeutic Environment. *International Journal of Therapeutic Communities*, 29: 228–244.

Pencheon, D. (2012). People and planet: from vicious cycle to virtuous circle. *British Medical Journal*, doi: 10.1136/bmj.e3774

Perrine, C. G., Sharma, A. J., Jefferds, M. E. D., Serdula, M. K. and Scanlon, K. S. (2010). Adherence to vitamin D recommendations among US infants. *Pediatrics*, 125: 627–632.

Phelan, J. C., Link, B. G., Stueve, A. and Pescosolido, B. A. (2000). Public conceptions of mental illness in 1950 and 1996: What Is mental illness and is it to be feared? *Journal of Health and Social Behavior*, 41(2): 188–207.

Phoenix Futures (n.d.). *Recovery through nature*. Online at: www.phoenix-futures.org.uk/our-services/recovery-through-nature/

Piff, P. K., Stancato, D. M., Côte, S., Mendoza-Denton, R. and Keltner, D. (2012). Higher social class predicts increased unethical behavior. *PNAS*, 109: 4086–4091.

Pitkala, K. H., Routasalo, P., Kautiainen, H. and Tilva, R. S. (2009). Effects of psychosocial group rehabilitation on health, use of health care services, and mortality of older persons suffering from loneliness: a randomised, controlled trial. *Journal of Gerontology: Medical Sciences*, 64A(7): 792–800.

Plotnikoff, R. C., Bercovitz, K. and Loucaides, C. A. (2004). Physical activity, smoking, and obesity among Canadian school youth: Comparison between urban and rural schools. *Canadian Journal of Public Health*, 95: 413–418.

Poloma, M. M. and Pendleton, B. F. (1991). The effects of prayer experiences on measures of general well-being. *Journal of Psychology and Theology*, 19(1), 71–83.

Powch, I. (1994). Wilderness Therapy: What makes it empowering for women? *Women and Therapy*, 15: 11–27.

Powell, K. E., Paluch, A. E. and Blair, S. N. (2011). Physical activity for health: What kind? How much? How intense? On top of what? *Annual Review of Public Health*, 32: 349–365.

Pratt, M., Sarmiento, O. L., Montes, F., Ogilvie, D., Marcus, B. H., et al. (2012). The implications of megatrends in information and communication technology and transportation for changes in global physical activity, *The Lancet*, 380(9838): 282–293.

Pretty, J. (2003). Social capital and the collective management of resources. *Science*, 302, 1912–1915.

Pretty, J. (2013). The consumption of a finite planet: well-being, convergence, divergence, and the nascent green economy. *Environmental and Resource Economics*, 55(4): 475–499.

Pretty, J. N. and Ward, H. (2001). Social capital and the environment. *World Development*, 29(2): 209–227.

Pretty, J., Peacock, J., Sellens, M. and Griffin, M. (2005). The mental and physical health outcomes of green exercise. *International Journal of Environmental Health Research*, 15: 319–337.

Pretty, J., Peacock, J., Hine, R., Sellens, M., South, N. and Griffin, M. (2007). Green exercise in the UK countryside: effects on health and psychological well-being, and implications for policy and planning. *Journal of Environmental Planning and Management*, 50: 211–231.

Pretty, J., Angus, C., Bain, M., Barton, J., Gladwell, V., et al. (2009). Nature, childhood, health and life pathways. *Interdisciplinary Centre for Environment and Society Occasional Paper 2009–02*. Online at: www.lotc.org.uk/wp-content/uploads/2011/04/Nature-Childhood-and-Health-iCES-Occ-Paper-2009-2-FINAL.-1-.pdf

Pretty, J., Barton, J., Colbeck, I., Hine, R., Mourato, S., Mackerron, G. and Wood, C. (2011). Health values from ecosystems. In *National Ecosystem Assessment*. London: Defra.

Pretty, J., Barton, J., Bharucha, Z. P., Bragg, R., Wood, C. and Pencheon, D. (2015). Improving health and well-being independently of GDP: dividends of greener and prosocial economies. *International Journal of Environmental Health Research*, 11: 1–26.

Price, D. B., Finniss, D. G. and Benedetti, F. (2008). A comprehensive review of the placebo effect: recent advances and current thought. *Annual Review of Psychology*, 59: 565–590.

Prince, M., Knapp, M., Guerchet, M., McCrone, P., Prina, M., et al. (2014). *Dementia UK: Update*. London: Alzheimer's Society.

Project Scotland (2014). *How it Works for Volunteers*. Online at: www.projectscotland.co.uk/volunteers/how-it-works/

Proper, K. I., Staal, B. J., Hildebrandt, V. H., van der Beek, A. J. and van Mechelen, W. (2002). Effectiveness of physical activity programs at worksites with respect to work-related outcomes. *Scandinavian Journal of Work, Environment and Health*, 28: 75–84.

Pryor, A., Carpenter, C. and Townsend, M. (2005). Outdoor education and bush adventure therapy: A socio-ecological approach to health and well-being. *Australian Journal of Outdoor Education*, 9: 3–13.

Pryor, A., Townsend, M., Maller, C. and Field, K. (2006). Health and well-being naturally: "contact with nature" in health promotion for targeted individuals, communities and populations. *Health Promotion Journal of Australia*, 17(2): 114–123.

Public Health England (2013a). *Obesity and the Environment: Increasing Physical Activity and Active Travel*. London: Public Health England.

Public Health England (2013b). *Social and Economic Inequalities in Diet and Physical Activity*. London: Public Health England.

Public Health England (2014). *National Child Measurement Programme Operational Guidance 2014*. Online at: www.gov.uk/government/uploads/system/uploads/attachment_data/file/308248/NCMP_updated_operational_guidance_02052014__3_.pdf

Public Health England (2015). *Public Health England "Identifying what works for local physical inactivity interventions"*. London: Public Health England.

Public Health, Plymouth City Council (2013). *Plymouth's National Child Measurement Programme (NCMP)*. Online at: www.plymouth.gov.uk/plymouths_national_child_measurement_programme.pdf

Putnam, R. (1995). Bowling alone: America's declining social capital. *Journal of Democracy*, 6(1): 65–78.

Puttick, R. and Ludlow, J. (2012). *Standards of Evidence for Impact Investing*. London: Nesta.

Pyle, R. M. (1978). The Extinction of Experience. *Horticulture*, 56: 64–67.

Pyle, R. M. (1993). *The Thunder Tree: Lessons from an Urban Wildland*. Boston: Houghton-Mifflin.

Pyle, R. M. (2001). The rise and fall of natural history: how a science grew that eclipsed direct experience. *Orion*, 20: 17–23.

Quinn, J. (2013). New learning worlds: the significance of nature in the lives of marginalised young people. *Discourse*, 34: 716–730.

Raanaas, R. K., Evensen, K. H., Rich, D., Sjostrom, G. and Patil, G. (2011). Benefits of indoor plants on attention capacity in an office setting. *Journal of Environmental Psychology*, 31: 99–105.

Rappe, E. and Kivela, S. L. (2005). Effects of garden visits on long-term care residents as related to depression. *HortTechnology*, 15(2), 298–303.

Rashid, M. and Zimring, C. (2008). A review of the empirical literature on the relationships between indoor environment and stress in health care and office settings—Problems and prospects of sharing evidence. *Environment and Behavior*, 40: 151–190.

Ratcliffe, E., Gatersleben, B. and Sowden, P. T. (2013). Bird sounds and their contributions to perceived attention restoration and stress recovery. *Journal of Environmental Psychology*, doi: 10.1016/j.jenvp.2013.08.004.

Razon, S., Basevitch, I., Land, W., Thompson, B. and Tenenbaum, G. (2009). Perception of exertion and attention allocation as a function of visual and auditory conditions. *Psychology of Sport and Exercise*, 10(6): 636–643.

Rea, T. and Waite, S. (2012). Issue 17: Are educational reform policies that stress standards and accountability compatible with pedagogical aims and practices in outdoor education? No. Taken Over? Schooling and Outdoor Education. In Martin, B. and Wagstaff, M. (eds), *Controversial Issues in Adventure Programming*. Champaign, IL.: Human Kinetics, pp. 265–271.

Reed, K., Wood, C., Barton, J., Pretty, J. N., Cohen, D. and Sandercock, G. (2013). A repeated measures experiment of green exercise to improve self-esteem in UK school children. *PloS one*, 8(7): e69176, doi: 10.1371/journal.pone.0069176

Retief, F. P. and Cilliers, L. (2006). The evolution of hospitals from antiquity to the Renaissance. *Acta Theologica Supplementum*, 7: 213–232.

Rew, K. (2008). *Wild Swim: River, Lake, Lido and Sea: The Best Places to Swim Outdoors in Britain*. London: Guardian Books.

Rickinson, M., Dillon, J., Teamey, K., Morris, M., Choi, M., et al. (2004). *A Review of Research on Outdoor Learning*. Shrewsbury: Field Studies Council.

Robinson, C. (2011). *Real World Research*. (3rd edn). Chichester: Wiley.

Rockstrom, J., Steffen, W., Noone, K., Persson, A., Chapin, F. S., et al. (2009). Planetary boundaries: exploring the safe operating space for humanity. *Ecology and Society*, 14(2): 32.

Roe, J. J., Ward Thompson, C., Aspinall, P. A., Brewer, M. J., Duff, E. I., et al. (2013). Green space and stress: Evidence from cortisol measures in deprived urban communities. *International Journal of Environmental Research and Public Health*, 10: 4086–4103.

Roe, J. and Aspinall, P. (2011). The restorative benefits of walking in urban and rural settings in adults with good and poor mental health. *Health and Place*, 17: 103–113.

Roemmich, J. N., Epstein, L. H., Raja, S., Yin, L., Robinson, J. and Winiewicz, D. (2006). Association of access to parks and recreational facilities with physical activity of young children. *Preventive Medicine*, 43: 437–441.

Rogers, C. R. (1951). *Client-centered Therapy: Its Current Practice, Implications and Theory*. Boston, MA: Houghton Mifflin.

Rogerson, M. and Barton, J. (2015). Effects of the visual exercise environments on cognitive directed attention, energy expenditure and perceived exertion. *International Journal of Environmental Research and Public Health*, 12(7): 7321–7336.

Rogerson, M., Brown, D., Sandercock, G., Wooler, J. and Barton, J. (2015). A comparison of four typical green exercise environments and prediction of psychological health outcomes. *Perspectives in Public Health*, doi: 10.1177/1757913915589845.

Roszak, T., Gomes, M. and Kanner, A. D. (eds) (1995). *Ecopsychology: Restoring the Earth, Healing the Mind*. San Francisco, CA: Sierra Club Books.

Royal College of Psychiatrists (2008). *Mental Health and Work*. London: Royal College of Psychiatrists.

Royal Society (2012). *People and the Planet*. London: Royal Society.

RSPB (2010). *Every Child Outdoors. Children need nature. Nature needs children*. Summary Report. Online at: www.rspb.org.uk/Images/everychildoutdoors_tcm9-259689.pdf

RSPB (2012). 'Disconnected children' mean nature is at risk. Online at: www.rspb.org.uk/media/releases/326839-disconnected-children-mean-nature-is-at-risk

Russell, K. C. (1999). *Theoretical Basis, Process and Reported Outcomes of Wilderness Therapy as an Intervention and Treatment for Problem Behaviour in Adolescents*. ID: College of Graduate Studies, University of Idaho.

Russell, K. C. (2001a). *Assessment of Treatment Outcomes in Outdoor Behavioural Healthcare*. ID: Wilderness Research Centre, University of Idaho.

Russell, K. C. (2001b). What is wilderness therapy? *Journal of Experiential Education*, 24(2): 70–79.

Russell, K. C. (2006a). Brat camp, boot camp, or....? Exploring wilderness therapy program theory. *Journal of Adventure Education and Outdoor Learning*, 6: 51–67.

Russell, K. C. (2006b). Evaluating the effects of the Wendigo Lake Expeditions program on young offenders. *Journal of Juvenile Justice and Youth Violence*, 4: 185–203.

Russell, K. C., Hendee, J. C. and Cooke, S. (1998). Potential Social and Economic Contributions of Wilderness Discovery as an Adjunct to the Federal Job Corps Program. *International Journal of Wilderness*, 4: 32–38.

Russell, K. C., Hendee, J. C. and Phillips-Miller, D. (2000). How wilderness therapy works: An examination of the wilderness therapy process to treat adolescents with behavioral problems and addictions. *Wilderness Science in a Time of Change Conference*, 3: 207–217.

Ryan, R. M., Weinstein, N., Bernstein, J., Brown, K. W., Mistretta, L. and Gagne, M. (2010). Vitalizing effects of being outdoors and in nature. *Journal of Environmental Psychology*, 30(2): 159–168.

Sallis, J. F., Prochaska, J. J. and Taylor, W. C. (2000). A review of the correlates of physical activity in children and adolescents. *Medicine and Science in Sports and Exercise*, 32: 963–975.

Samson, C. and Pretty, J. (2006). Environmental and health benefits of hunting lifestyles and diets for the Innu of Labrador. *Food Policy*, 31(6): 528–553.

Sandercock, G., Angus, C. and Barton, J. (2010). Physical activity levels of children living in different built environments. *Preventive Medicine*, 50: 193–198.

Schiffman, S. S., Suggs, M. S. and Sattely-Miller, E. A. (1995). Effect of pleasant odors on mood of males at midlife: comparison of African-American and European-American men. *Brain Research Bulletin*, 36: 31–37.

Schultz, P. W. (2002). Inclusion with nature: The psychology of human-nature relations. In Schmuck, P. and Schultz, W. P. (eds), *Psychology of sustainable development*. Norwell, MA: Kluwer. pp. 62–78.

Schultz, S. E., Kleine, R. E. and Kernan, J. B. (1989). "These Are a Few of My Favourite Things". Toward an explication of attachment as a consumer behavior construct. *Advances in Consumer Research*, 16: 359–366.

Searles, H. (1960). *The Nonhuman Environment: In Normal Development and Schizophrenia*. New York: International Universities Press.

Sebba, R. (1991). The landscapes of childhood. *Environment and Behavior*, 23(4): 395–422.

Sempik, J. (2007). *Researching Social and Therapeutic Horticulture for People with Mental Ill Health: a study of methodology*. Reading and Loughborough: Thrive and Centre for Child and Family Research (CCFR).

Sempik, J. and Aldridge, J. (2006). Care farms and care gardens: Horticulture as therapy in the UK. In Hassink, J. and van Dijk, M. (eds), *Farming for Health: green-care farming across Europe and the United States of America*. New York: Springer.

Sempik, J. and Bragg, R. (2013). Green Care: Origins and Approaches. In Gallis, C. (ed.), *Green Care: for Human Therapy, Social innovation, Rural Economy, and Education*. New York: Nova Science Publishers.

Sempik, J., Aldridge, J. and Becker, S. (2003). *Social and Therapeutic Horticulture: Evidence and Messages from Research*. Reading and Loughborough: Thrive and Centre for Child and Family Research (CCFR).

Sempik, J., Aldridge, J. and Becker, S. (2005). *Health, Wellbeing and Social Inclusion, Therapeutic Horticulture in the UK*. Bristol: The Policy Press.

Sempik, J., Hine, R. and Wilcox, D. (eds) (2010). *Green Care: a conceptual framework, a report of the working group on the health benefits of Green Care, COST Action 866, Green care in Agriculture*. Loughborough: Centre for Child and Family Research, Loughborough University.

Shanahan, D. F., Fuller, R. A., Bush, R., Lin, B. B. and Gaston, K. J. (2015). The Health Benefits of Urban Nature: How Much Do We Need? *BioScience*, 65(5): 476–485.

Shapiro, S. L., Oman, D., Thoresen, C. E., Plante, T. G. and Flinders, T. (2008). Cultivating mindfulness: effects on well-being. *Journal of Clinical Psychology*, 64(7): 840–862.

Sherman, E. and Newman, E. S. (1977). The meaning of cherished personal possessions for the elderly. *Journal of Aging and Human Development*, 8: 181–192.

Sherwood, N. E. and Jeffery, R. W. (2000). The behavioral determinants of exercise: implications for physical activity interventions. *Annual Review of Nutrition*, 20(1): 21–44.

Sheu-Jen, H., Wen-chi, H., Patricia, S. and Jackson, P. W. (2010). Neighbourhood environment and physical activity among urban and rural schoolchildren in Taiwan. *Health and Place*, 16: 470–476.

Shibata, S. and Suzuki, N. (2004). Effects of an indoor plant on creative task performance and mood. *Scandinavian Journal of Psychology*, 45(5): 373–381.

Simpson, K. A. and Singh, M. A. (2008). Effects of exercise on adiponectin: a systematic review. *Obesity*, 16: 241–256.

Staats, H., and Hartig, T. (2004). Alone or with a friend: A social context for psychological restoration and environmental preferences. *Journal of Environmental Psychology*, 24(2): 199–211.

Stamatakis, E. and Chaudhury, M. (2008). Temporal trends in adults' sports participation patterns in England between 1997 and 2006: the Health Survey for England. *British Journal of Sports Medicine*, doi: 10.1136/bjsm.2008.048082

Stepping Stones to Nature (2012). *Annual Report Year 3 July 2011-June2012*. Online at: www.plymouth.gov.uk/ss2nannual_report.pdf

Sternberg, E. (2009). *Healing Spaces*. Cambridge, MA: Harvard University Press.

Stewart, A. (2008). Whose place, whose history? Outdoor environmental education pedagogy as 'reading' the landscape. *Journal of Adventure Education and Outdoor Learning*, 8(2): 79–98.

Sugiyama, T., Leslie, E., Giles-Corti, B. and Owen, N. (2008). Associations of neighbourhood greenness with physical and mental health: Do walking, social coherence and local social interaction explain the relationships? *Journal of Epidemiology and Community Health*, 62(9), doi: 10.1136/jech.2007.064287

Sullivan, W. C. (2015). In search of a clear head. In Kaplan, R. and Basu, A. (eds), *Fostering Reasonableness: Supportive Environments for Bringing Out Our Best*. Ann Arbor, MI: University of Michigan Press, pp. 54–69.

Suttie, J. (1984). Wilderness: A medium for Improving Psychological Health. *The Environmentalist*, 4: 295–299.

Takano, T., Nakamura, K. and Watanabe, M. (2002). Urban residential environments and senior citizens' longevity in megacity areas: the importance of walkable green spaces. *Journal of Epidemiology and Community Health*, 56: 913–918.

Tapsell, S., Tunstall, S., House, M., Whomsley, J. and Macnaghten, P. (2001). Growing up with rivers? Rivers in London children's worlds. *Area*, 33: 177–189.

Taylor, A. F. and Kuo, F. E. (2009). Children with attention deficits concentrate better after walk in the park. *Journal of Attention Disorders*, 12(5): 402–409.

Taylor, A. F., Kuo, F. E. and Sullivan, W. C. (2001). Coping with ADD: The surprising connection to green play settings. *Environment and Behaviour*, 33: 54–77.

Taylor, A. F., Kuo, F. E. and Sullivan, W. C. (2002). Views of nature and self-disciple: Evidence from inner city children. *Journal of Environmental Psychology*, 22: 49–64.

Teas, J., Hurley, T., Ghumare, S. and Ogoussan, K. (2007). Walking outside improves mood for healthy postmenopausal women. *Clinical Medicine: Oncology*, 1: 35–43.

Tennessen, C. M. and Cimprich, B. (1995). Views to nature: Effects on attention. *Journal of Environmental Psychology*, 15: 77–85.

Thoits, P. A. and Hewitt, L. N. (2001). Volunteer work and well-being. *Journal of Health and Social Behavior*, 42: 115–131.

Thompson, S. and Kent, J. (2014). Connecting and strengthening communities in places for health and well-being. *Australian Planner*, 51(3): 260–271.

Thompson Coon, J., Boddy, K., Whear, R., Barton, J. and Depledge, M. H. (2011). Does participating in physical activity in outdoor natural environments have a greater effect on mental well-being than physical activity indoors? A systematic review. *Environmental Science and Technology*, 45: 1761–1772.

Thompson, J.E.S., Webb, R., Hewlett, P., Llewellyn, D. and Mcdonnell, B. (2013). Matrix metalloproteinase-9 and augmentation index are reduced with an 8-week green-exercise walking programme. *Journal of Hypertension*, 2: 127.

Tighe, M., Whiteford, A. and Richardson, J. (2013). Stepping Out: Enabling community access to green space through interdisciplinary practice learning in Plymouth, UK. *International Journal of Practice-based Learning in Health and Social Care*, 1(2): 8–22.

Timperio, A., Giles-Corti, B., Crawford, D., Andrianopoulos, N., Ball, K., et al. (2008). Features of public open spaces and physical activity among children: Findings from the CLAN study. *Preventive Medicine*, 47: 514–518.

Tops, M., van Peer, J. M., Korf, J., Wijers, A. A. and Tucker, D. M. (2007). Anxiety, cortisol, and attachment predict plasma oxytocin. *Psychophysiology*, 44: 444–449.

Townsend, M. and Ebden, M. (2006). *Feel Blue, Touch Green*, Final Report. Melbourne: Deakin University. Online at: www.deakin.edu.au/__data/assets/pdf_file/0006/310749/Feel-Blue,-Touch-Green.pdf

Townsend, M. and Moore, M. (2005). *Research into the Health, Well-being and Social Capital Benefits of Community Involvement in the Management of Land for Conservation*, Final Report. Melbourne: Deakin University.

Townsend, M. and Weerasuriya, R. (2010). *Beyond Blue to Green: the Benefits of Contact with Nature for Mental Health and Wellbeing*. Online at: www.hphpcentral.com/wp-content/uploads/2010/09/beyondblue_togreen.pdf

Townsend, M., Henderson-Wilson, C., Warner, E. and Weiss, L. (2015). *Healthy parks, healthy people: the state of the evidence 2015*. Melbourne: Deakin University.

Trost, S. G., Kerr, L., Ward, D. S. and Pate, R. R. (2001). Physical activity and determinants of physical activity in obese and non-obese children. *International Journal of Obesity*, 25: 822–829.

Trost, S. G., Owen, N., Bauman, A. E., Sallis, J. F. and Brown, W. (2002). Correlates of adults' participation in physical activity: review and update. *Medicine and Science in Sports and Exercise*, 34: 1996–2001.

Tsai, Y. M., Chou, S. W., Lin, Y. C., Hou, C. W., Hung, K. C., et al. (2006). Effect of resistance exercise on dehydroepiandrosterone sulfate concentrations during a 72-h recovery: relation to glucose tolerance and insulin response. *Life Sciences*, 79: 1281–1286.

Tsunetsugu, Y, Park, B.-J., Ishii, H., Hirano, H., Kagawa, T. and Miyazaki, Y. (2007). Physiological Effects of Shinrin-yoku (Taking in the Atmosphere of the Forest) in an Old-Growth Broadleaf Forest in Yamagata Prefecture, Japan. *Journal of Physiological Anthropology*, 26: 135–142.

Tsunetsugu, Y., Park, B.-J. and Miyazaki, Y. (2010). Trends in research related to "Shinrin-yoku" (taking in the forest atmosphere or forest bathing) in Japan. *Environmental Health and Preventive Medicine*, 15: 27–37.

Tsunetsugu, Y., Park, B.-J., Lee, J., Kagawa, T. and Miyazaki, Y. (2011). Psychological relaxation effect of forest therapy: Results of field experiments in 19 forests in Japan involving 228 participants. *Japanese Journal of Hygiene*. 66: 670–676.

Tuan, Y. F. (1977). *Sense and Place*. Minneapolis, MN: University of Minnesota Press.

Tudor-Locke, C. (2010). Steps to better cardiovascular health: how many steps does it take to achieve good health and how confident are we in this number? *Current Cardiovascular Risk Reports*, 4: 271–276.

Tuke, D. H. (1882). *Chapters in the History of the Insane in the British Isles*, first published London 1882, reprinted 1968, Amsterdam: E. J. Bonset.

Tunstall, S. and Penning-Rowsell, E. (1998). The English Beach: Experiences and Values. *The Geographical Journal*, 164: 319–332.

Tunstall, S., Tapsell, S. and House, M. (2004). Children's perceptions of river landscapes and play: what children's photographs reveal. *Landscape Research*, 29: 181–204.

Twenge, J. M. Baumeister, R. F., DeWall, C. N., Ciarocco, N. J. and Bartels, J. M. (2007). Social exclusion decreases prosocial behavior. *Journal of Personality and Social Psychology*, 92(1): 56–66.

Twiss, J., Dickinson, J., Duma, S., Kleinman, T., Paulsen, H. and Rilveria, L. (2013). Community gardens: lessons learned from California healthy cities and communities. *American Journal of Public Health*, 93: 1435–1438.

UNEP (2011). Towards a Green Economy: Pathways to Sustainable Development and Eradication of Poverty. Nairobi: UNEP.

Union of Concerned Scientists (2014). *The $11 Trillion Reward. How Simple Dietary Changes Can Save Lives and Money, and How We Can Get There*. Cambridge, MA: Union of Concerned Scientists.

Ulrich, R. S. (1981). Natural versus urban scenes: some psychophysiological effects. *Journal of Environment and Behaviour*, 13: 523–556.

Ulrich, R. S. (1984). View through a window may influence recovery from surgery. *Science*, 224: 420–421.

Ulrich, R. S. (1993). Biophilia, biophobia and natural landscapes. In Kellert, S. R., Wilson, E. O. (eds), *The Biophilia Hypothesis*. Washington D.C.: Island Press.

Ulrich, R. S. (2002). *Health Benefits of Gardens in Hospitals*. Paper for conference, Plants for People International Exhibition Floriade.

Ulrich, R. (2008). Biophilic Theory and Research for Healthcare Design. In Kellert, S. R., Heerwagen, J. and Mador, M., *Biophilic Design: The Theory, Science, and Practice of Bringing Buildings to Life*. Hoboken, NJ: Wiley.

Ulrich, R. S., Simons, R. F., Fiorito, E., Miles, M. A. and Zelson, M. (1991). Stress recovery during exposure to natural and urban environments. *Journal of Environmental Psychology*, 11: 201–230.

UNCRC (United Nations Convention on the Rights of the Child). (1989). *Convention on the Rights of the Child*. Online at: http://media.education.gov.uk/assets/files/pdf/u/uncrc%20%20%20full%20articles.pdf

UNICEF (2012). *Levels and Trends in Child Mortality*. New York: UNICEF.

USDA ERS (2013). *Food availability (per capita) data system*. Online at: www.ers.usda.gov/data-products/food-availability-(per-capita)-data-system.aspx

Van den Berg, A. E., Maas, J., Verheij, R. A. and Groenewegen, P. P. (2010). Green space as a buffer between stressful life events and health. *Social Science and Medicine*, 70: 1203–1210.

Vecchio, R. P. (1980). The function and meaning of work and the job: Morse and Weiss (1955) revisited. *Academy of Management Journal*, 23: 361–367.

Veitch, J., Salmon, J., Carver, A., Timperio, A., Crawford, D., et al. (2014). A natural experiment to examine the impact of park renewal on park-use and park-based physical activity in a disadvantaged neighbourhood: the REVAMP study methods, *BMC Public Health*, 14: 600, doi: 10.1186/1471-2458-14-600

Verderber, S., (1986). Dimensions of person-window transactions in the hospital environment. *Environment and Behaviour*, 18: 450–466.

Villanueva, K., Giles-Corti, B., Bulsara, M., Timperio, A., McCormack, G., et al. (2013). Where do children travel to and what local opportunities are available? the relationship between neighbourhood destinations and children's independent mobility. *Environment and Behavior*, 45(6): 679–705.

Visit England (2012). *The GB Day Visitor: Statistics 2011*. Edinburgh: TNS.

Waddell, G. and Burton A. K. (2006). *Is Work Good for your Health and Well-being?* London: The Stationery Office.

Waite, S. (2010). Losing our way?: Declining outdoor opportunities for learning for children aged between 2 and 11. *Journal of Adventure Education and Outdoor Learning*, 10(2): 111–126.

Waite, S. (2013). 'Knowing your place in the world': how place and culture support and obstruct educational aims. *Cambridge Journal of Education*, 43(4): 413–434.

Waite, S. (2014). *Natural Connections and Outdoor Learning in the UK/England*. Paper presented at symposium, National Institute of Education, Nanyang Technical University, Singapore.

Waite. S. (2015). Culture clash and concord: supporting early learning outdoors in the UK. In Prince, H., Henderson, K. and Humberstone, B. (eds), *International Handbook of Outdoor Studies*. London: Routledge.

Waite, S. and Pleasants, K. (2012). Cultural Perspectives on Experiential Learning in Outdoor Spaces. *Journal of Adventure Education and Outdoor Learning*, 12(3): 161–165.

Waite, S. and Pratt, N. (2015). Situated learning (Learning in Situ). In Wright, J. D. (ed.), *International Encyclopaedia for the Social and Behavioural Sciences*, 2nd edition, Vol. 22. Oxford: Elsevier.

Walker, S. (2011). *The Spirit of Design*. London: Earthscan.

Walter, P. (2013). Greening the Net Generation: Outdoor Adult Learning in the Digital Age, *Adult Learning*, 24(4): 151–158.

Walters, G. (1998). *Changing Lives of Crime and Drugs. Intervening with substance-abusing offenders*. New York: Wiley.

Walton, J. (2000). *The British Seaside: Holidays and resorts in the twentieth century*. Manchester: Manchester University Press.

Wapner, S., Demick, J. and Redondo, J. P. (1990). Cherished possessions and adaptation of older people to nursing homes. *International Journal of Aging and Human Development*, 31(3): 219–235.

Ward, T. and Maruna, S. (2007). *Rehabilitation: beyond the risk paradigm*. London: Routledge.

Ward Thompson, C., Aspinall, P. and Montarzino, A. (2008). The childhood factor: adult visits to green places and the significance of childhood experiences. *Environment and Behaviour*, 401: 111–143.

Ward Thompson, C., Roe, J. and Aspinall, P. (2013). Woodland improvements in deprived urban communities: What impact do they have on people's activities and quality of life? *Landscape and Urban Planning*. 118: 79–89.

Ward Thompson, C., Roe, J., Aspinall, R., Mitchell, R., Clow, A. and Miller, D. (2012). More green space is linked to less stress in deprived communities; evidence from salivary cortisol patterns. *Landscape and Urban Planning*, 105: 221–229.

Warr, P. B. (1987). *Work, Unemployment and Mental Health*. Oxford: Oxford Science Publications.

Wattchow, B. and Brown, M. (2011). *A Pedagogy of Place: outdoor education for a changing world*. Clayton: Monash University Publishing.

Welk, G. J., Blair, S. N., Wood, K., Jones, S. and Thompson, R. W. (2000). A comparative evaluation of three accelerometry-based physical activity monitors. *Medicine and Science in Sports and Exercise*, 32: S489–497.

Wells, N. and Lekies, K. S. (2006). Nature and the life course: pathways from childhood nature experiences to adult environmentalism. *Children, Youth and Environments*, 16: 1–24.

Wells, N. and Rollings, K. (2012). The natural environment: influences on human health and function. In Clayton, S. (ed.), *The Oxford Handbook of Environmental and Conservation Psychology*. London: Oxford University Press.

Wells, N. M., Ashdown, S. P., Davies, E. H. S., Cowett, F. D. and Yang, Y. (2007). Environment, design and obesity. Opportunities for interdisciplinary collaborative research. *Environment and Behaviour*, 39: 6–33.

Wheeler, B. W., White, M., Stahl-Timmins, W. and Depledge, M. H. (2012). Does living by the coast improve health and wellbeing? *Health and Place*, 18: 1198–1201.

White, R. and Heerwagen, J. (1998). Nature and mental health: Biophilia and Biophobia. In Lundberg, A. (ed.), *The Environment and Mental Health: A guide for clinicians*. Bergen County, NJ: Lawrence Erlbaum Associates.

White, M., Smith, A., Humphryes, K., Pahl, S., Snelling, D. and Depledge, M. (2010). Blue space: the importance of water for preference, affect and restorativeness ratings of natural and built scenes. *Journal of Environmental Psychology*, 30(4): 482–493.

White, M. P., Hignett, A. and Pahl, S. (2011). Surf to Success: Can Learning to Surf Promote Individual and Environmental Well-Being? A Preliminary Assessment of Global Boarders' Surf to Success Programme. *ECOMINDS*.

White, M., Alcock, I., Wheeler, B. and Depledge, M. (2013a). Would you be happier living in a greener urban area? A fixed-effects analysis of panel data. *Psychological Science*, 23: 920–928.

White, M. P., Alcock, I., Wheeler, B. W. and Depledge, M. H. (2013b). Coastal proximity, health and well-being: Results from a longitudinal panel survey. *Health and Place*, 23: 97–103.

White, M. P., Pahl, S. Ashbullby, K. J., Herbert, S. and Depledge, M. H. (2013c). Feelings of restoration from recent nature visits. *Journal of Environmental Psychology*, 35: 40–51.

White, M. P., Wheeler, B. W., Herbert, S., Alcock, I. and Depledge, M. H. (2014). Coastal proximity and physical activity: Is the coast an under-appreciated public health resource? *Preventive Medicine*, 69C: 135–140.

Whitelaw, S. (2012). The emergence of a "dose–response" analogy in the health improvement domain of public health: A critical review. *Critical Public Health*, 22: 427–440.

Whiteley, S. (2004). The Evolution of the Therapeutic Community. *Psychiatric Quarterly*, 75(3): 2332–47.

Whitzman, C., Worthington, M. and Mizrachi, D. (2009). *Walking the Walk: Can Child Friendly Cities Promote Children's Independent Mobility?* Melbourne: GAMUT [Australasian Centre for the Governance and Management of Urban Transportation].

Wichstrom, L., von Soest, T. and Kvalem, I. L. (2013). Predictors of growth and decline in leisure time in physical activity from adolescence to adulthood. *Health Psychology*, 32(7): 775–784.

Wickramasekera, N., Wright, J., Elsey, H., Murray, J. and Tubeuf, S. (2015). Cost of crime: a systematic review. *Journal of Criminal Justice*, 43: 218–228.

Wilkinson, R. and Marmot, M. (2003). *The Solid Facts: Social Determinants of Health*, (2nd edn). Copenhagen: World Health Organization.

Williams, B. (2000). The treatment of adolescent populations: an institutional vs. a wilderness setting. *Journal of Child and Adolescent Group Therapy*, 10(1): 47–56.

Williams, M. and Penman, D. (2011). *Mindfulness*. London: Pitakus.

Williams, D. M., Dunsiger, S., Ciccolo, J. T., Lewis, B. A., Albrecht, A. E. and Marcus, B. H. (2008). Acute affective response to a moderate-intensity exercise stimulus predicts physical activity participation 6 and 12 months later. *Psychology of Sport and Exercise*, 9(3): 231–245.

Wilson, E. O. (1986). *Biophilia: the human bond with other species*. Cambridge, MA: Harvard University Press.

Wilson, S. J. and Lipsey, M. W. (2000). Wilderness challenge programs for delinquent youth: a meta-analysis of outcome evaluations. *Evaluation and Planning*, 23: 1–12.

Windhager, S., Atzwangera, K., Booksteina, F. and Schaefera, K. (2011). Fish in a mall aquarium–An ethological investigation of biophilia. *Landscape and Urban Planning*, 99: 23–30.

Witten, K., Hiscock, R., Pearce, J. and Blakely, T. (2008). Neighbourhood access to open spaces and the physical activity of residents: a national study. *Preventive medicine*, 47: 299–303.

Wood, C. (2012). *Exercise environment and physical activity in children and adolescents*. Colchester: University of Essex.

Wood, C., Bragg, R., Pretty, J. and Barton, J. (2012a). *The TurnAround Project- Phase 3*. Colchester: The Wilderness Foundation, University of Essex.

Wood, C., Bragg, R., Pretty, J. and Barton, J. (2012b). *The Health Benefits of the 'Generations Growing Together' (GGT)*. Colchester: University of Essex.

Wood, C., Angus, C., Pretty, J., Sandercock, G. and Barton, J. (2013a). A randomised control trial of physical activity in a perceived environment on self-esteem and mood in UK adolescents. *International Journal of Environmental Health Research*, 23(4): 311–320.

Wood, C., Bragg, R. and Barton, J. (2013b). *The TurnAround Project- Phase 4*. Colchester: The Wilderness Foundation, University of Essex.

Wood, C., Gladwell, V. and Barton, J. L. (2014a). A repeated measures experiment of school playing environment to increase physical activity and enhance self-esteem in UK school children. *Plos One* 9(9): e108701, doi: 10.1371/journal.pone.0108701

Wood, C., Sandercock, G. and Barton, J. L. (2014b). Interactions between physical activity and the environment to improve adolescent psychological well-being: a randomized controlled trial. *International Journal of Environment and Health*, 7(2): 144–155.

Wood, M., Cattell, J., Hales, G., Lord, C., Kenny, T. and Capes, T. (2015). *Re-offending by offenders on Community Orders Results from the Offender Management Community Cohort Study*. Ministry of Justice, Online at: https://www.gov.uk/government/uploads/system/uploads/attachment_data/file/399388/reoffending-by-offenders-on-community-orders.pdf

World Health Organization (WHO) (1948). Preamble to the Constitution of the World Health Organization as adopted by the International Health Conference. 19–22 June 1946, New York.

World Health Organization (2010). *Global Recommendations on Physical Activity for Health*. Geneva: World Health Organization. Online at: http://www.ncbi.nlm.nih.gov/books/NBK305057/pdf/Bookshelf_NBK305057.pdf

World Health Organization (2010). *WHO Report: Global status report on noncommunicable diseases 2010: Description of the global burden of NCDs, their risk factors and determinants*. Geneva: World Health Organisation.

WWF (2010). *Living Planet Report*. London and Oakland: WWF and Global Footprint Network.

WWF (2012). *China ecological footprint record 2012*. London and Oakland: WWF and Global Footprint Network.

Xavier, S. and Mandal, S. (2005). The psychosocial impacts of obesity in children and young people: A future health perspective. *Public Health Medicine*, 6: 23–27.

Yamaguchi, M., Deguchi, M. and Miyazaki, Y. (2006). The effects of exercise in forest and urban environments on sympathetic nervous activity of normal young adults. *Journal of International Medical Research*, 34: 152–159.

Yamashita, S. (2002). Perception and evaluation of water in landscape: use of Photo-Projective Method to compare child and adult residents' perceptions of a Japanese river environment. *Landscape and Urban Planning*, 62(1): 3–17.

Yanagisawa, H., Dan, I., Tsuzuki, D., Kato, M., Okamoto, M., et al. (2010). Acute moderate exercise elicits increased dorsolateral prefrontal activation and improves cognitive performance with stroop test. *Neuroimage*, 50: 1702–1710.

Yerkes, R. M. and Dodson, J. D. (1908). The relation of strength of stimulus to rapidity of habit formation. *Journal of Comparative Neurology and Psychology*, 18: 459–482.

Zak, P. J., Stanton, A. A. and Ahmadi, S. (2007). Oxytocin increases generosity in humans. *PLoS ONE*, 2(11): e1128.

Zeisel, J. (2009). *I'm Still Here: a breakthrough approach to understanding someone living with Alzheimer's*. New York: Penguin.

Zube, E. H., Pitt, D. G. and Evan, G. W. (1983). A lifespan developmental study of landscape preference. *Journal of Environmental Psychology*, 3: 115–128.

Zubieta, J.-K. and Stohler, C. S. (2009). Neurobiological mechanisms of placebo responses. *Annals of New York Academy of Science*, 1156: 198–210.

Index

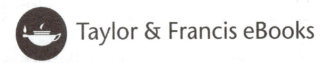